HEALING
HERBS
A to Z

A HANDY REFERENCE
TO HEALING PLANTS

HEALING
HERBS

A TO Z

Diane Stein

CROSSING PRESS
Berkeley | Toronto

Crossing Press
A division of Ten Speed Press
PO Box 7123
Berkeley CA 94707
www.tenspeed.com

Distributed in Australia by Simon and Schuster Australia, in Canada by
Ten Speed Press Canada, in New Zealand by Southern Publishers Group,
in South Africa by Real Books, and in the United Kingdom and Europe by
Publishers Group UK.

Cover design and interior design by theBookDesigners

Library of Congress Cataloging-in-Publication Data
Stein, Diane, 1948-
Healing herbs A to Z : a handy reference to healing plants / Diane Stein.
p. ; cm.
Includes index.
ISBN-13: 978-1-58091-192-4 (alk. paper)
ISBN-10: 1-58091-192-7 (alk. paper)
1. Herbs—Therapeutic use. 2. Medicinal plants. 3. Materia medica,
Vegetable. I. Title.
[DNLM: 1. Plants, Medicinal. 2. Phytotherapy. QV 766 S819h 2009]
RM666.H33.S74 2009
615'.321—dc22

2008030058

First printing, 2009

Printed in Canada

1 2 3 4 5 6 7 8 9 10 — 13 12 11 10 09

The material presented here is for information and educational purposes
only, and is not meant to take the place of expert or medical advice. The
information in this book does not intend to diagnose, cure, or treat disease.
Individual reactions to herbs may vary. In situations of illness, seek the
professional help of your choice.

CONTENTS

INTRODUCTION

In 1985 when I wrote *The Women's Spirituality Book* (now titled *Diane Stein's Guide to Goddess Craft*), I wanted to include a chapter on using herbs. At that time, I had been working with herbs for a few years and was very excited about it, but I felt I didn't know enough to write even a chapter on them. When I wrote *All Women Are Healers* five years later, I got a little braver and did an herb chapter. After twenty-five years of studying and using herbs and making my own tinctures, I am finally compiling an herbal, as I have always wanted to do. I still feel that I don't know enough and could never know enough—but that I have to start where I am and hope the real experts will be indulgent with my effort.

This book is not designed for herbal experts, though they may find useful information here. This book is for the confused layperson who wants to regain control of her health but doesn't know where to start.

The first thing an herb user needs to know is which herb will do what she needs. The second is to find the herb and identify it accurately (a mistake in the field can be toxic or even fatal). And the third is to know how to use the herb appropriately. A traditional herbalist learns from those who know how to use herbs, information that used to be passed down from teacher to student, or from mother to daughter, over many generations through ancient and time-honored oral tradition. She learns how to recognize herbs accurately, along with when to pick them, and which plant parts to harvest and use. She also learns how and when to use them—and when not to.

Tragically, that oral tradition has been lost. Most of us who wish to learn about herbs do so from books, the Internet, or by taking a workshop here and there, followed by limited experience with personal use.

Traditional herbalists used what was growing in the neighboring woods and fields, and locally harvested herbs were considered the most useful for people living in that area. But this limited the number and variety of plants available. Today's herb users have many more plant varieties available to them from all over the United States, South America, Europe, Africa, and Asia.

For those who choose herbal healing, the way to do it may not be to go to the woods and fields to identify, pick, and process the right local plants. It may simply mean a visit to the local health food store, natural pharmacy, or herb website to buy what's needed.

This book is a reference guide for the herb shopper who, while not having the benefit of ancient oral tradition or personal instruction, still wants to use herbs as knowledgeably as she can.

Herbs used properly are very often as effective as medical drugs—or more so—without the side effects, cost, and potential for dependency. Herbs help people become enabled, instead of disabled. They leave us stronger, not weaker. But we need to learn how and when to use them, as well as when to seek more expert help, which might mean consulting a physician, midwife, or acupuncturist. We need to understand the appropriate uses of herbs—for example, when it's safe to substitute black cohosh for hormone replacement therapy (which for many of us presents an unacceptable risk of cancer) to treat the uncomfortable symptoms of menopause.

This book is intended for the herb shopper, not the professional practitioner. It explains what's in the bottles lined up on the shelves of the local health food store and the conditions that each herb helps heal. The information is presented in a highly concentrated way—not pages of explanation and description, but a quick reference of the herb's primary attributes and uses. Where a more comprehensive herbal reference book might also describe how to identify the plant, where to find it, when to pick it, which parts to use, and how to prepare those parts, this book assumes that the user will buy already identified, prepared, and ready-to-use plant material. Dosages and dosing instructions (how many drops or capsules, how many times a day) are listed on the bottle, along with how long the herb can be used safely, and contraindications for its use.

Ready-prepared herbs come in several forms. Traditional use is as an herb tea, called a **tisane**, or the harder-boiled tea, called a **decoction**, for preparing woody plant parts, which may be ingested or applied externally in a **compress** (wet a cloth with the tea or decoction and place it on the body) or a **poultice** (wrap the boiled herb matter in a cloth and place it on the body). Herbs also come in capsules, which are easy to take but may be less effective than ingesting a tea or decoction, because the raw, dried herbs in them may not be as fresh and harder for the body to assimilate. Some herbs also come in salves, creams, or ointments for external use only.

Another frequently found form for internal use is the **tincture** or **extract**, where the herb is steeped cold in alcohol (brandy, vodka) for several weeks. The herb matter is then strained out, and the alcohol, which has extracted the herb's benefits, is used medicinally. To remove the alcohol from an alcohol extract, put the drops of herb preparation in a few teaspoons of boiling or near-boiling water and the alcohol will evaporate in a few seconds, leaving the potency of the herb.

Alcohol-free glycerin tinctures are also available and are often used for children or by those who do not wish to ingest alcohol. Glycerin is sugar, however. It does not keep as long or as bacteria-free as alcohol preparations, is not as medicinally strong, and is not safe for diabetics.

The one herbal usage to avoid, for the purposes of this book, is the **essential oil**. This is an entirely different branch of healing, where the oils from some plants are distilled into a highly concentrated form. Essential oils are not to be taken internally, as they can be highly toxic and even result in death with just a few drops. They are used externally, and the healing benefits come from inhaling their fragrances. If you are interested in this form of healing, there are many books on aromatherapy (the use of essential oils) to get you started. For external use, only the essential oils of lavender and tea tree may be used directly on the skin. All others must be diluted, usually one drop of oil to a teaspoon of "carrier oil," generally a vegetable salad oil.

The few oils found in this book are the **essential fatty acids** and meant for ingestion—evening primrose oil, flaxseed oil, borage oil, sea buckthorn oil, black currant oil—and they come in capsules for that purpose. Wild oregano oil needs to be diluted, and sometimes comes that way. These are not essential oils, and no essential oil is to be taken internally without the direction of an aromatherapy expert.

Essential oils, by the way, are not the same as **flower essences** (also known as essential essences), which are the vibrations of flowers preserved in alcohol or a vinegar tincture. Flower essences are not discussed here, but refer to my book *Healing with Flower and Gemstone Essences* for more on their use.

The information in this book focuses on using one herb at a time. Single herbs used alone are traditionally called "simples." Experienced herbalists often use several herbs together, but for those who are learning, it's less confusing and more important to learn what each herb does before combining them. Some commercial herbal combinations may contain a dozen or more herbs, which to me seems to miss the point. If you want to understand how herbs work, you must do it one herb at a time. Also, not all herbs work well together. It's best to use them individually until you gain experience.

Read labels for warnings and possible drug interactions. If you are taking any medications, their effects can be increased, decreased, altered, or deactivated by a particular herb. It is very important to research your medications' interactions with *any* herb you are considering. (For example, blood thinners, such as the anticoagulant warfarin, are contraindicated due to potentially dangerous interaction.) The Internet has made this relatively easy to do, but be aware that there are a number of websites whose main purpose seems to be to scare people away from using herbs altogether. Herbs used properly are safe, but it is essential to make informed decisions.

With each herb entry, I have included information on side effects, warnings, and possible drug interactions. In some cases it has been very difficult to separate fact from fiction on this subject. For the most part, herb side effects happen only with misuse, overuse, or contaminated herbs. Some side effects are simply the effects of the herb itself. Increased sweating or diarrhea, for example, may be among the herb's uses, one of the ways the herb works for healing. Most toxic side-effect disasters are caused by ingestion of essential oils *that were never meant to be ingested*. It is important to realize, too, that each person is different, and how an herb reacts for you may be slightly different from another person's reactions to it. Also, anyone can be allergic to anything, whether peanuts or goji juice. Obviously, if you have an allergic reaction to an herb, or any other disquieting effect, *stop taking it*. I have tried to responsibly list as many drug interactions and side effects as possible, but my information cannot be considered complete; there are thousands of medications available, with more being added daily.

For acute conditions, such as a cold or sore throat, expect the right herb for the condition to begin having benefit after two or three doses, sometimes sooner. For chronic conditions, such as menstrual difficulties or arthritis, it will usually take longer. Some herbs (and conditions) can take as long as two or three months for the benefits to become evident. So be patient, and adjust your expectations. Healing often occurs gradually, and you may experience more improvement than you realize at first.

If you have a serious dis-ease—I use this form of the word to note that we are not "diseased" but may have "lack of ease" in our bodies—it is best to seek professional advice for it. Whether this means advice from a physician, an herbalist, or another kind of healer, that is your choice. If you choose to use herbs for serious conditions, it is wise to seek the advice of an experienced herbalist.

This is also the case if you wish to have herbal support in pregnancy or for an abortion. Some of the herbs in this book are designated safe for pregnancy and some are not. Those that are listed as not for use in pregnancy or nursing may be acceptable with the advice of a skilled herbalist or midwife. Many herbs are labeled "not for pregnancy or breastfeeding" simply to err on the side of caution. Some herbs listed in this book are abortifacients; they bring on menses that can cause an abortion early in pregnancy. Although the information belongs to women and adamantly needs to be available, herbs should not be used to replace a professional medical procedure in a sanitary clinical setting.

There is a list of specialized terms that herbalists frequently use, each one indicating an herb's attributes and providing a shorthand description of what the herb does. An experienced herbalist looks at the list and immediately knows how to use the herb. Sources often differ on the attributes assigned to an herb. In this book, I have tried to reconcile various sources, and in cases where an herb has no research list, I have attempted to assign one. I have also attempted to make it a list that is understandable to nonherbalists. For example, an herb listed as an "emmenogogue" (classic definition: brings blood flow to the pelvic area and uterus) may be described as a uterine toner or "brings on menses." I have done my best with these terms. For a version of the classic list, see below.

I hope this book will be a convenient reference for those who wish to learn about using herbs. Even more, I hope it will help those who need healing and are looking for safe alternatives to drugs. Herbs link the past, present, and future of human life; they are a vital part of our herstory.

UNDERSTANDING
THE MEDICINAL ATTRIBUTES OF HERBS

Adaptogen – tonic, normalizes all systems and organs, stress healer

Alterative – changes assimilation processes to regulate body functions

Analgesic – pain reliever

Antibacterial – kills or prevents bacterial growth

Anticatarrhal – eliminates mucus (*see* Expectorant)

Anticoagulant – blood thinner

Antiemetic – stops or relieves vomiting

Antifungal – kills or prevents the growth of fungi

Antihistamine – reduces or stops allergic reactions

Anti-inflammatory – stops or reduces inflammation

Antimicrobial – kills or reduces the spread of all microscopic pathogens (bacteria, fungi, viruses, parasites)

Antiparasitic – kills or prevents the growth of parasites (intestinal worms, protozoa, amoeba, etc.)

Antipyretic – lowers body temperature to reduce fevers

Antiseptic – kills toxic bacteria to prevent infection

Antispasmodic – calms contraction of smooth muscles; for twitching, spasms, coughing, cramping

Antiviral – kills or prevents the growth of viruses

Aphrodisiac – increases libido and sexual function

Aromatic – fragrant, spicy herbs that stimulate the gastrointestinal system

Astringent – contracts, constricts, or shrinks tissues, stops discharges

Carminative – eases digestive cramps and releases gas

Cholagogue – stimulates secretion of bile

Demulcent – soothes and provides a protective coating

Diaphoretic – causes sweating to break a fever

Diuretic – increases urination, eliminates excess water from the body

Emetic – causes vomiting

Emmenagogue – increases blood flow to the uterus and pelvis

Expectorant – thins and expels respiratory tract mucus

Hepatic – regulates bile

Hormonal – plant with hormonal properties, phytoestrogen

Laxative – stimulates bowel movements

Mucilaginous – expands and adheres to tissues to soothe them

Nervine – benefits the nervous system, nerve tonic, calms the nerves

Sedative – central nervous system depressant, calms and relaxes

Stimulant – increases the action of the body or of a specific system or organ

Stomachic – improves stomach function, increases appetite

Tonic – strengthens and tones organs and systems

Vermifuge – expels intestinal worms

Vulnerary – heals wounds

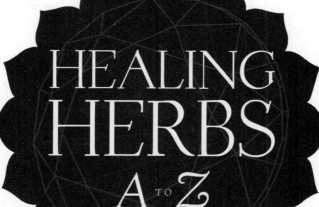

HEALING
HERBS
A TO Z

HERB
LISTINGS

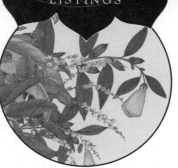

HERB LISTINGS

Alfalfa • *(Medicago sativa)*

Grass native to Iran in the Bronze Age, planted for animal feed and as a nitrogen soil fixative worldwide; more a food plant than a medicinal herb but also used medicinally; high in minerals and vitamins, amino acids, protein, enzymes, iron, and chlorophyll, good protein source for vegetarians; tonic, detoxifier, liver and blood cleanser, pituitary stimulant, glandular balance; diuretic for fluid retention, swelling, edema, kidney stones, bladder and kidney infections, rheumatoid arthritis, lumbago, prostate enlargement, jaundice; used for stomach disorders, all types of ulcers, colitis, to help increase appetite, listed by some sources as a cure for diabetes; used externally as a poultice for black-and-blue bruises, wounds, joint pain, and muscle pain; bath herb, facial steam, hair rinse. Reduces high fevers, reduces bleeding, helps blood clot, lowers high blood pressure, lowers cholesterol; antiviral, clears infections, clears grass allergies, aids drug and alcohol withdrawal, laxative, provides vitamins and nutrients to aid and prevent night blindness; good in pregnancy to prevent bleeding, increases breast milk, reduces tooth decay, promotes healthy teeth and bones in mother and child, prevents anemia, strengthens children that fail to thrive and grow, strengthens connective tissue; combine white willow, burdock, and alfalfa for a tasty arthritis tea. *Nutrient, tonic, appetite stimulant, diuretic.* No known side effects; avoid with gout and lupus, overuse of alfalfa can induce lupus in susceptible people; allergy potential if allergic to peas, soy, or peanuts; may interfere with diabetic drugs, diuretics, blood thinners (anticoagulants).

All Heal • *See* Self Heal

Aloe Vera • (Also known as *Aloe barbadensis*)
Use in topical gel or 2 to 4 ounces of juice drunk daily; juice has almost no taste and is most effective when a tablespoon of liquid chlorophyll is added; also used during colonic treatments; effective for all skin irritations and dis-eases, burns,

4

radiation burns, sunburn, boils, insect bites, athlete's foot, poison ivy and oak, wounds, cuts, acne, eczema, psoriasis, ringworm, dark spots on skin, scalp and hair damage and dis-eases; skin moisturizer and cell regenerator; heals gum dis-ease and mouth canker sores (rinse with liquid); use as a gargle for sore throat and tonsillitis; prevents infection, helps bronchial congestion, antiseptic and tissue-soothing for cystitis and kidney infection, detoxifies; drink juice to heal internal ulcers (ulcerative colitis, ulcerative bowel dis-eases, and stomach ulcers); best remedy for constipation, bowel regularity, intestinal irritations and dis-eases, inflammatory bowel diseases, hemorrhoids, heartburn, upset stomach, reduces toxic flora in intestines and yeast overruns, liver damage, detoxifies and cleanses the entire digestive system, aid for weight loss and loss of appetite; heals the uterus and brings on menses, can be used as a douche; helps joint and muscle strain and pain, especially after hard exercise; increases protein absorption; immune enhancer, tonic; increases general energy and feelings of well-being; reduces triglycerides, reduces total cholesterol, increases good HDL cholesterol; high in minerals, vitamins, and amino acids. *Anti-inflammatory, antioxidant, astringent, diuretic, liver tonic, laxative, wound healer.* Possible side effects: cramps, diarrhea, laxative dependence; do not use with abdominal pain (possible appendicitis), avoid in pregnancy and breastfeeding.

Angelica • *(Angelica archangelica, Angelica officinalis)*
Garden angelica, also called wild celery; not the Chinese angelica (dong quai); expectorant to clear infections with lung congestion: colds, cough, flu, pleurisy, bronchitis, pneumonia, whooping cough, asthma; can be used as a chest poultice; strengthens digestion, reduces gas, colic, heartburn, gastritis, appetite loss, anorexia nervosa; increases blood sugar levels; regulates the menstrual cycle, helps restore cycles after going off the Pill, brings on menses, eases menstrual cramps, PMS, mood swings, water retention, and contracts the uterus; immune stimulant; diuretic and urinary antiseptic for cystitis, gout, rheumatism; reduces fever by sweating; calms the nerves; aids weakness, debility, and recovery after illness; warms the body, stimulates circulation especially to the extremities; use for cold hands and feet, Buerger's dis-ease (narrowed arteries in hands and feet), neuralgia. *Expectorant,*

astringent, diuretic, digestive stimulant, antibacterial, antiviral, antifungal, tonic. Possible side effects: contact dermatitis; not for use in pregnancy or breastfeeding, by diabetics, with heart dis-ease, or when taking blood thinners. Oil is never to be used internally; safe short term but may cause photosensitivity; not for use in the eyes.

Artichoke Leaf • *(Cynara scolymus)*

Related to milk thistle and with similar function, do not confuse with Jerusalem artichoke; major use is for promoting optimal liver function, which in turn reduces indigestion and high cholesterol; liver detoxifier, stimulates bile flow, opens obstructed bile ducts, prevents gallstones, antioxidant liver protector, aids insufficient liver function, aids liver regeneration, inhibits cholesterol production, stimulates breakdown and elimination of cholesterol; used for symptoms of nonspecific liver insufficiency, including fatigue, headache, lassitude, abdominal pain, bloating, nausea, constipation or diarrhea, heartburn, discomfort after meals, inability to eat foods with fat, increased allergies and sensitivities; used for inflamed liver, jaundice, hepatitis, cirrhosis, excessive use of alcohol, fatty liver; protects from liver damage; cleanses and protects the liver from pollutants, chemicals, alcohol; also lowers blood sugar levels (diabetes); facilitates function in kidney dis-ease, irritable bowel syndrome; normalizes bowel peristalsis, prevents viral replication in HIV and cancer, aids indigestion, anemia; lowers triglycerides, helps prevent heart dis-ease, may prevent DNA damage. *Antioxidant, liver protective, bile stimulant.* Not for use with gallstones or obstructed bile ducts, in pregnancy or breast-feeding; possible side effects: allergic reactions, gas, skin rash; no listed warnings or drug interactions.

Ashwaganda • *(Withania somnifera)*

Adaptogen similar in properties to Korean ginseng, used for thousands of years in India, also called winter cherry; used alone and in many herbal combinations; normalizes healthy whole body function when challenged by stress; supports adaptation to stress, resistance to dis-ease and aging; promotes better physical and mental performance; nourishes the brain, muscles, bones, and endocrine system; promotes immune function; also is antioxidant, rejuvenator, tonic, anti-inflammatory, sexual enhancer; prevents some cancers and tumors; enhances mental function for memory, mood, clarity, alertness, concentration, and focus; aids debility, anxiety, depression, exhaustion, adrenal exhaustion, mental and physical fatigue including stress-induced fatigue, chronic fatigue, insomnia; also used for arthritis, rheumatism, ulcers, swollen glands, colds, cough, flu, bronchitis, inflamed eyes, anemia, infertility, gynecological disorders, aging, and to induce general feeling of vitality and wellness. *Adaptogen, anti-inflammatory, antitumor, antioxidant, antistress.* No toxicity but may cause drowsiness; overdose causes restlessness; best when taken only a few days a week, or take for three weeks and stop for the fourth; should not be used in pregnancy or breastfeeding; increases the effects of other herbs and drugs (expert advice recommended).

Astragalus • *(Astragalus membranaceus)*

Used in traditional Chinese medicine for immune enhancement, immune balancing, and all auto-immune dis-eases; safe used long term; delicious as a tea or in soup; use for all immune dis-eases, chronic fatigue, CMV (cytomegalovirus), HIV and AIDS, HPV (human papilloma virus, cervical cancer, vaginal warts), tuberculosis, lupus; anticancer, may increase effectiveness of chemotherapy, reduces chemotherapy side effects (especially fatigue, appetite loss) and genital herpes; asthma, multiple allergies, long-standing infections, stomach ulcers, arthritis; increases white blood cell count, supports the adrenals; useful for critical dis-eases including stroke, heart dis-ease, heart inflammation, high blood pressure, high cholesterol, improves heart function, kidney dis-ease and failure, liver dis-ease and hepatitis B and C, diabetes (reduces blood sugar levels), diabetes leg and foot ulcers, diabetic neuropathy, hyperthyroidism; also for viral infections (colds, flu), upper respiratory infections, fever, anemia, wound healing, burn healing, indigestion (diarrhea, gas, bloating, colic), irregular menstruation, menstrual disorders, insomnia, diuretic, tonic; enhances athletic performance, increases mental acuity in children, possible help in Alzheimer's dis-ease and dementia, aids in stopping smoking. *Antiviral, immune enhancer, anticancer, antifungal, anti-inflammatory, antimicrobial, antioxidant.* Few or no side effects but large overdose can suppress the immune system; okay for children if they do not have a fever; may increase the effects of antiviral drugs, diabetes drugs, blood pressure drugs, blood thinners, diuretics; may counteract immune-depressant drugs like cyclosporine.

Bacopa • *(Bacopa monnieri)*
Ayurvedic herb, also called water hyssop; benefits mind, spirit, and consciousness; used to consecrate and "awaken" newborns; tonic that supports and enhances brain and mental function, cognitive function, increases intelligence, short- and long-term memory, alertness, mental clarity, learning, information retention, concentration; used for neurodegenerative dis-eases, such as Alzheimer's dis-ease, ADHD and restlessness in children, senility of aging, mental disorders, forgetfulness, depression, students' learning aid; relaxant, mildly sedative, antianxiety, antiseizure; cardio tonic, digestive aid, improves respiratory function, thyroid stimulant, protects the liver from drug damage, reduces fats in blood; free-radical antioxidant; rejuvenates; reduces allergies and allergic reactions for asthma, hay fever, eczema; protects the gastrointestinal tract lining and decreases smooth muscle spasms for indigestion, ulcers, irritable bowel syndrome; laxative; inhibits

cancer growth; also for anemia, fevers, bronchitis, bronchial constriction, antifungal for *Candida albicans*. *Antioxidant, vasodilator, anticancer, sedative, antifungal, antimicrobial.* No listed side effects; long-term use is needed for benefit; may decrease effectiveness of thyroid drugs and increase effects of sedatives.

Barberry • *(Berberis vulgaris)*

The root and bright red berries of the prickly hedge, used since ancient Egypt as a medicinal; can be substituted for Oregon grape root or goldenseal; stimulant and cleanser for the liver, normalizes liver function, promotes bile flow, clears jaundice, reduces enlarged liver and spleen; digestive bitter, indigestion, heartburn; treats bacterial, fungal, and viral infections, kills *Pseudomonas* bacteria, *E. coli, Streptococcus,* and other bacteria in the body: bacterial diarrhea, traveler's dysentery, food poisoning, urinary tract infections, respiratory infections (sore throat, lung and nasal congestion, sinusitis, bronchitis, conjunctivitis), skin infections and dis-eases; intestinal parasites, yeast overrun; also used for gout and rheumatism, abnormal uterine bleeding, fever, convulsions, appetite stimulant, immune stimulant, sedative; lowers blood pressure by dilating blood vessels; may shrink tumors. *Antibacterial, antifungal, antiviral, antiparasitic, astringent, anti-inflammatory, antibiotic, laxative, bitter tonic.* Overdose side effects include diarrhea, nosebleed, vomiting, dizziness, confusion, drop in blood pressure, kidney dis-ease; not for use in pregnancy or breastfeeding, or for infants; not for those with heart or chronic respiratory diseases; use short term only; may increase or decrease the effects of some medical drugs.

Bee Propolis, Bee Pollen • *See* Propolis

Beet Root • *(Beta vulgaris)*
Properties of sugar beet (or borscht beet) are long known to juicers—juicing is still the best way to utilize the benefits; blood purifier, regenerates red blood cells, high in iron, regulates blood pH balance, heals acidosis, heals anemia, replaces blood loss in menstruating women, raises low blood sugar, increases energy and vitality, and oxygenates the body through the blood; detoxifies the liver, gallbladder, spleen, and kidneys; clears obstructions from liver and spleen; for

liver dis-eases, jaundice, hepatitis, cirrhosis, biliousness, liver toxicity from alcohol, constipation and diarrhea, dysentery, hemorrhoids; promotes bowel peristalsis; inhibits formation of tumors, growths, and cancer cells; promotes resistance to cancer, dissolves cancer cells and tumors; reduces tumors of lung, prostate, breast, and uterus; promising antiviral for HIV/AIDS; lowers high blood pressure, lowers total and LDL cholesterol to prevent heart dis-ease and strokes; skin detoxifier used internally and as a poultice to draw out toxins, for acne, boils, abscesses, scabs, skin infections and inflammations, measles and children's eruptive dis-eases, dandruff; also for varicose veins, ulcers, fever, swollen glands, sore throat, viral and bacterial infections, resistance to infections and dis-ease, and as an aphrodisiac. *Anticancer, antitumor, liver protective, detoxifier.* A nutritious food, no known warnings, cautions, or drug interactions; take care not to overuse and detoxify too quickly; start with very small amounts and increase gradually, cut back if uncomfortable; red urine from beet ingestion is harmless.

Bilberry • *(Vaccinium myrtillus)*

Relative to the blueberry plant, used medicinally by Hildegard of Bingen (1098–1179); active ingredients are anthocyanosides, strong antioxidants, also high in vitamin C; protects, heals, and regenerates the capillaries, increases capillary circulation, reduces blood clots, relaxes all the blood vessels of the circulatory system; stops bleeding, prevents easy bruising, lowers risk of heart attacks and strokes, reduces high blood pressure, lowers triglycerides, lowers cholesterol, lowers blood sugar, regenerates connective tissue, and protects against cancer (antiangiogenesis); for peripheral vascular dis-eases: improves night vision, reduces or reverses degenerative eye dis-eases, macular degeneration, glaucoma, cataracts, diabetic retinopathy, eyestrain, myopia, retinitis pigmentosa; varicose veins, spider veins, swollen legs, chronic venous insufficiency, Raynaud's syndrome, Bell's palsy, emphysema, hemorrhoids, fibrocystic breast dis-ease; also for chronic inflammatory diseases, gastrointestinal dis-eases, diarrhea, dysentery, food poisoning, peptic ulcers (inhibits *H. pylori* bacteria), blood in stool or urine, bleeding gums; liver dis-eases, gallstones, kidney disease; inflamed mucous membranes, respiratory viruses, sore

throat, fevers, skin infections and ulcers, wounds; diuretic for
cystitis, rheumatoid arthritis, gout, rheumatism, and painful
menstruation; prevents or stops production of breast milk.
*Antioxidant, diuretic, astringent, anti-inflammatory, vascular
protective.* Considered a food and very safe, no side effects with
normal use; overdose effects include indigestion, nausea, and
diarrhea; safe in pregnancy but may stop breast milk if nursing; caution with diabetes drugs (bilberry lowers blood sugar),
blood thinners, antiulcer drugs, and laxative drugs.

Bitter Melon • *(Momordica charantia)*
Known and used in India, Asia, South America, Africa, and
the Caribbean as an insulin substitute for the treatment of
diabetes; regulates blood sugar, works by suppressing the
neural response to sweet-taste stimuli, increases production
of beta cells in the pancreas, regulates carbohydrate metabolism, increases cell uptake of glucose, raises insulin levels
in the blood, increases effectiveness of diabetic medications;
also reduces high blood pressure, high cholesterol, high triglyceride levels; stimulates digestion, lowers body temperature,
reduces inflammation, detoxifies, raises immune function, is

contraceptive, may help prevent HIV replication, and may be effective against leukemia and a variety of cancers; used for many illnesses and dis-eases: constipation, mucus conditions, fevers, colds and coughs, flu, hemorrhoids, jaundice, intestinal worms and parasites, indigestion, acute gastritis, poor digestion, malaria, chronic fatigue, ulcers, skin conditions, sores and wounds; increases breast milk, and regulates hormones. *Antibacterial, antioxidant, antimicrobial, astringent, antispasmodic, antiviral, hypoglycemic.* Possible side effects: diarrhea or indigestion; diabetics need to monitor blood sugar levels carefully with any antidiabetic herb or drug; not for use in pregnancy or breastfeeding, or if wanting to get pregnant; not for those with hypoglycemia.

Blackberry • *(Rubus fructicosus, Rubus species)*
Delicious in tea and easily available in any supermarket; active ingredient is tannin, an herbal astringent; primarily used for diarrhea and sore throat; for diarrhea, dysentery, food poisoning, hemorrhoids, bowel inflammations, intestinal ulcers; inflammation of throat, mouth, gums; tightens loose teeth; common cold with sore throat, laryngitis, tonsillitis, lung dis-

eases, bronchitis; loosens phlegm; also reduces heavy menstrual flow, brings on menses, corrects lack of menses; uterine tonic, douche for vaginitis; eases labor pain; skin tonic and for all skin conditions (used externally), boils, eczema; black hair dye; traditionally used for whooping cough, appendicitis, and cholera; diuretic for swollen feet and ankles (kidney and heart dis-ease), gout, swollen arthritic joints, rheumatism, cystitis; poison antidote, antidote for venomous snakebites and insect bites; anemia; antioxidant to prevent and reverse cell damage, preventive for heart dis-ease, cancer, strokes, degenerative eye dis-eases such as cataracts and macular degeneration. *Anti-inflammatory, astringent, tonic, mild diuretic, stops bleeding.* A very few sensitive individuals may experience nausea or vomiting, especially those with chronic gastrointestinal dis-ease; no known drug interactions.

Black Cohosh • *(Cimicifuga racemosa)*

Primary herb for menopause relief, safe alternative to hormone replacement therapy, including after hysterectomy; not an estrogen and with no estrogenic effects; can be taken long term, takes several weeks before benefits manifest; menopause

18

relief for hot flashes, night sweats, bloating, breast swelling and cystic breasts, osteoporosis (slows or prevents bone loss), weight gain, fatigue, mood swings, anxiety, depression, irritability, hormone imbalance, insomnia, memory loss, headaches and migraines, fibroids, vaginal dryness, heart palpitations, high blood pressure, menstrual cramps, PMS, cervical dysplasia, heavy periods, painful periods, inflammations of uterus and ovaries, and most gynecological disorders (these uses are for women of all ages if needed); used in younger women for infertility, endometriosis, threatened miscarriage, to induce labor, labor pain relief, heavy periods, PMS, cystic breasts, ovarian cysts, fibroid tumors, hormone imbalance, cervical dysplasia, painful periods, heavy bleeding in menstruation, and other gynecological conditions; other uses include mild sedative, neurological conditions, kidney infections, gallbladder and liver, malaria, rheumatism, arthritis and joint pain, hives, back pain, coughs, colds, fever, tinnitus, appetite stimulant, diuretic, diarrhea. *Astringent, diuretic, expectorant, menstrual tonic, antispasmodic, sedative.* Do not overdose; mild side effects may include headache, indigestion, weight gain, nausea, dizziness, sweating, and heaviness in the legs; rarely,

side effects may include nausea, indigestion, dizziness, headache, or sweating; not for use in pregnancy or nursing without
expert advice, not for those with liver dis-ease; increases the
effectiveness of the breast cancer drug tamoxifen; not estrogenic and does not foster breast cancer growth.

Black Currant Seed Oil • *(Ribes nigrum)*
Used interchangeably with flaxseed oil for its essential fatty
acids, including gamma-linolenic acid (GLA) and omega-3
and omega-6 fatty acids. *See* Flaxseed Oil for more uses; primarily used for heart support and protection against heart
attack and stroke, prevents blood clots, reduces inflammation in the circulatory system, regulates heart rate; lowers
blood pressure and cholesterol levels, dilates the blood vessels, lowers triglycerides, aids sodium-potassium balance
in the body; also used as an anti-inflammatory for the pain
and swelling of joint dis-eases (arthritis, rheumatoid arthritis), PMS, menopausal symptoms, sinusitis, and as a tumor
and cancer preventive; normalizes gastrointestinal function,
heart function, cardiovascular function, allergic response,
hormone and steroid production, neurological and brain

function, bone support; immune enhancer especially for the elderly, raises T-cell function and production, enhances resistance to bacterial and viruses; protects the pancreas and pancreatic function; diabetes support; heals the skin and hair, protects the body from stress; effective as antiaging. *Antiinflammatory, antitumor, anticancer, diuretic.* Considered safe even long term, the only listed side effect is diarrhea; not recommended for hemophiliacs, those taking blood thinner drugs, or in pregnancy without expert advice.

Black Haw • *(Viburnum prunifolium)*

Used interchangeably with cramp bark (*Viburnum opulus*); but black haw was used primarily by white and Native American colonial-era women for the uterus; also used by slave owners to prevent black slave women from aborting unwanted pregnancies; relaxes muscles by blocking the enzyme that causes spasms; useful for every muscle in the body (internal and external), every discomfort resulting from muscle spasms and overcontraction, and every pain associated with movement; use for muscle pain and tension, cramps of all kinds (menstrual, uterine, muscle cramps, stomach or intestinal cramps), irritable bowel syndrome, constipation, headache, contracted muscles in arthritis, joint pain, back pain, pain of mumps and swollen glands, lockjaw; menstrual and menopausal pain and blood loss; brings on delayed or too light menses, stops threatened miscarriage or abortion, hormonal migraines, endometriosis; sedative, calms and soothes the nerves, nervous tension, nervous disorders, seizures; lowers blood pressure, heart palpitations, improves blood circulation, circulatory dis-eases, heart dis-ease; rheumatism, breathing difficulties, asthma, colic. *Antispasmodic, anti-inflammatory, astringent, sedative.* Little research has been done on this traditional herb; no known side effects; may worsen tinnitus, no known drug interactions.

Black Walnut Hulls • *(Juglans nigra)*

Blood purifier and detoxifier known to the ancient Greeks and Romans; used externally and internally as a vermifuge, antifungal, and antiseptic; use topically and internally together for all blood and intestinal parasites, and for all toxic blood conditions: ringworm, pinworm, tapeworm, fungus infections, vaginal infections (douche), *Candida albicans*, coccidia, giardia, warts, herpes, cold sores, poison ivy, poison oak, scrofula, impetigo, tuberculosis, venomous bites, hair loss, dandruff, athlete's foot, nail fungus, syphilis, jock itch; all skin dis-eases with sores, wounds, bruising, acne, eczema, psoriasis, hemorrhoids, tumors, mouth sores, ulcers, boils, abscesses, tumors; laxative but also heals diarrhea, lowers high blood pressure, cleanses blood vessels of cholesterol, lowers LDL cholesterol, lowers blood sugar, dissolves kidney stones; induces healthy sleep patterns, builds teeth, strengthens muscles and nerves, high in iodine for thyroid deficiency; also used for sore throats, tonsillitis, malaria, coughs, asthma, chronic bronchitis, nosebleeds; digestion, colic, gas, heartburn, appetite loss; intestinal dis-eases, inflamed conditions of the bowel, colitis, ballooned or relaxed colon, rheumatism, gout, prolapsed uterus, brain disorders, glandular deficiencies and dis-eases, eye disorders and conjunctivitis; also stimulates liver bile, heals the spleen. *Astringent, antifungal, antiparasitic, antiseptic, anti-inflammatory, laxative.* May be toxic to kidneys and liver in overdose, stains the skin; should not be used with coughs with fever, when pregnant or breastfeeding; no known drug interactions.

Blessed Thistle • *(Cnicus benedictus)*

Not to be confused with milk thistle; used in the Renaissance as an all-healer where it was believed to prevent all sicknesses including plague; usually combined with other herbs; may be useful for eating disorders and appetite loss, including anorexia nervosa; stimulates breast milk production, brings on menses, stimulates menstrual flow, relieves menstrual pain, amenorrhea (lack of menses); detoxifier and disinfectant for cervical dysplasia, vaginal infections (douche), used in breast enhancement formulas; contraceptive and abortifacient; stimulates stomach acid and saliva; digestive bitter, indigestion, gas, gastrointestinal infections and dis-eases; liver stimulant, hepatitis, jaundice, headaches from liver congestion, bile flow, liver dis-eases, gallbladder dis-ease; anti-inflammatory, prevents and heals infections, antibacterial for some bacterial types, anticancer, stops bleeding, blood purifier, diuretic, fever (promotes sweating), enhances memory; clears respiratory mucus for colds, bronchitis; use topically for infections, skin ulcers, boils, wounds, gangrenous skin conditions, acne, and aids repair of collagen for skin healing. *Antioxidant, astringent, expectorant, diuretic, anti-inflammatory, digestive bitter, antibacterial, tonic.* Considered safe when used short term; side effects include allergy, stomach irritation, vomiting; not for use in pregnancy, with inflammatory bowel conditions, stomach ulcers, hiatus hernia, gastroesophageal reflux dis-ease; not recommended for use with blood thinners, aspirin or ibuprofen (NSAIDS), or antacids (including over-the-counter preparations).

Blue Cohosh • *(Caulophyllum thalictroides)*

Midwife's remedy used in the last two to three weeks of pregnancy and in labor for easy labor and delivery; induces labor, stimulates contractions, coordinates contractions, increases strength of contractions, prevents or stops false labor pains, prevents premature delivery and miscarriage, restarts stalled or inefficient labor, aids in delivering the placenta, stops bleeding after birth, reduces after-pains, eases restlessness in pregnancy, uterine tonic; use for PMS, menstrual cramps, chronic or acute uterine pain and inflammation, chronic or acute ovarian pain and inflammation, endometriosis, metritis, breast pain, vaginal infections, chlamydia, thrush, cervical dysplasia, for menopausal symptoms and pain; use to bring on menses and to regulate menstrual cycle; restores cycles after stopping birth control pills; abortifacient in very early pregnancy, especially used in tinctures with black cohosh and pennyroyal (never the oil); also used for rheumatism, arthritis inflammation, colic, bronchitis, pneumonia, whooping cough, asthma, bladder and kidney infections, gout, dropsy, sore throat, hiccups, epilepsy, muscle spasms of all kinds; calms nerves, improves memory. *Antispasmodic, diuretic, antibiotic, immune stimulant, vasodilator, uterine tonic, estrogenic.* Unless for abortion, take only in the last month of pregnancy, never in the first or second trimester; don't overuse; can cause headaches, nausea, high blood pressure, pains in arms and legs; powder can irritate skin and mucous membranes; avoid with estrogenic conditions and cancers; no known drug interactions.

Boldo • *(Peumus boldus, Peumus boldus molina)*
Kept handy in most South American households as a culinary spice and to stop indigestion; sold as tea bags in most Spanish supermarkets; stimulates the liver, gallbladder, and gastrointestinal tracts, protects and detoxifies, dissolves fats and relieves inflammation and pain; digestive bitter that

stimulates secretion of stomach juices; used for indigestion, dyspepsia, gas, stomach cramps, heartburn, ulcers, laxative, lack of appetite, and weight loss; stimulates bile for liver ailments, gallstones, fatty liver, jaundice, hepatitis; slows digestion in the intestines; use for intestinal cramps, spastic colon, inflammatory bowel dis-eases; expels parasites and worms; reduces uric acid production for gout and rheumatism; diuretic for bladder and kidney inflammation; use for cystitis, water retention, prostate enlargement; also tones the heart, increases blood flow to the heart, reduces heart rate, relaxes the blood vessels, inhibits blood clots; cellular protector and antioxidant, mild sedative; used for severe pain, insomnia, dizziness, to treat sexually transmitted infections, malaria, colds, earaches. *Anti-inflammatory, antioxidant, tonic, antiseptic, stimulant, diuretic, sedative.* No listed side effects; use only ascaridole-free preparations; not for long-term use, never take the essential oil internally; not for use in pregnancy or breastfeeding, with obstructed bile ducts or serious liver or kidney dis-ease; do not use with blood thinner drugs or aspirin; may reduce effectiveness of drugs that are processed by the liver.

Boneset • *(Eupatorium perfoliatum)*

Known by Native Americans and taught to the earliest colonists; written about by Avicena (980–1037 CE), aspirin substitute, primarily used for flu with body pain; standard herbal for colds, coughs, flu, bronchitis, upper respiratory congestion, sore throats, fever, minor viral dis-eases, chills, aches and pains, upset stomach; cold and flu preventive when taken at first symptoms; causes heavy sweating to break fever; decongestant, laxative; used for malaria and dengue (breakbone) fever, typhoid, cholera, pneumonia; anticonvulsive used for epilepsy and fever seizures; immune stimulant, increases white blood cell production; circulatory stimulant, digestive bitter, and liver tonic; diuretic for edema, water retention, urinary and kidney infections, gout; appetite stimulant, expels intestinal worms, snakebite remedy; use for gonorrhea, calming; aids digestion and indigestion in elderly people, heals body pain from many sources (arthritis, rheumatism); anti-inflammatory used topically for skin dis-eases and infected sores; regulates menstrual cycle, eases pain in childbirth; use warm or hot tea for flu symptoms; drink a cup every half hour or hour for three or four doses until sweating begins; use cool

28

tea as a general tonic. *Stimulant, laxative, reduces fevers, anti-spasmodic.* Do not eat the fresh leaves (liver toxic); not for use longer than two weeks, do not overdose or overuse (can cause vomiting and severe diarrhea); avoid in pregnancy; no known drug interactions; effective and safe.

Borage • *(Borago officinalis)*

Primarily used in capsules as an oil (pressed seeds, not essential oil); the plant leaves and stems may be liver toxic in large doses; food plant, contains omega-6 essential fatty acids for promoting heart and artery health; regulates hormone production and balance; glandular balancer, normalizes the metabolism; adrenal tonic for recovery from stress or surgery, and recovery of adrenal function after use of steroids or cortisone; known for its healing of menopausal symptoms, hot flashes, PMS, mood swings; increases breast milk after childbirth; significant anti-inflammatory action for arthritis, rheumatoid arthritis, rheumatism, joint damage and pain, also for inflammatory bowel dis-eases (such as irritable bowel syndrome, Crohn's dis-ease, colitis, diverticulitis), and skin disorders; expectorant for respiratory viruses, colds, flu, dry cough, sore throat, pleurisy, bronchitis, asthma; lowers fever by promoting sweating; heals the skin (external and internal use) for eczema, psoriasis, dermatitis, seborrhea, itching, swelling, healthy skin and nails, healthy hair; diuretic for kidney and bladder dis-eases, cystitis, kidney stones and urinary gravel, soothes and releases water retention; heals gastritis, cures hangovers; calming, sedative, reduces depression; stabilizes mood, nervous disorders, agitation, irritability, pain relief; reduces high blood pressure, high cholesterol, high triglycerides, relaxes the blood vessels to prevent heart dis-ease, heart attacks, and strokes. *Anti-inflammatory, diuretic, expectorant, vasodilator.* Oil side effects include belching, bloating, diarrhea, leaking of oil from rectum; the plant (not the oil) may be toxic in overdose; avoid in pregnancy, with seizure disorders, or if taking blood thinners (including aspirin).

Boswellin • *(Boswella serrata)*
Ayurvedic remedy made from the gum resin of the frankincense tree, active ingredient is boswellic acid, used internally and as a warming topical cream. Major anti-inflammatory action, especially for arthritis but throughout the body internally

and externally; protects tissues from inflammation damage, increases circulation to joints and tissues, and prevents deterioration of cartilage; used for arthritis (all types), rheumatism, aches and pains, muscle and joint pain, back pain, sports injuries; inflammatory bowel dis-eases such as chronic ulcerative colitis, Crohn's dis-ease, dysentery, bowel ulcers; lowers cholesterol and triglycerides, stimulates the thyroid, promotes hair growth and weight loss, relieves pain; immune balancer; also used for asthma, coughs, sores, snakebite, laryngitis, vomiting, fevers, abscesses; antitumor and anticancer properties, especially for brain tumors, inhibits leukemia; sedative, offers a sense of wellness and well-being. *Anti-inflammatory, antitumor, immune modulator, expectorant.* Mild side effects may include diarrhea, nausea, skin rash, heartburn, or aftertaste; no known warnings or drug interactions.

Burdock • *(Artium lappa)*

Good-tasting food herb especially pleasant in soups, high in fiber, minerals, and vitamins, including vitamin C; blood purifier and detoxifier used in Essiac, Hoxsey formula, as well as other anticancer and antiarthritis herbal combinations;

scientific research on burdock use for cancer, HIV, and bacterial infections is so far inconclusive; reduces blood sugar and may be helpful for diabetes; used for all skin and hair dis-eases (internally and externally), including hair loss, dandruff, itching scalp, sores, psoriasis, eczema, hives, lice and ringworm, warts, skin ulcers, acne, boils, bruises, burns, bites, and skin lesions that don't heal; diuretic for kidney stones, bladder and kidney infections, water retention; liver dis-eases, hemorrhoids, rheumatism, gout; colds, sore throat, fever, indigestion, sciatica; blood thinner, stomach toner, anti-inflammatory, laxative, relaxant, soothes all tissues; use for arthritis with alfalfa and white willow in a tasty tea. *Blood purifier, diuretic, induces perspiration, digestive bitter.* No known side effects but allergic reactions are possible, avoid if allergic to ragweed; may increase dehydration and hypoglycemia, or effects of drugs that are diuretic or lower blood sugar.

Butcher's Broom • *(Ruscus aculeatus)*

Used internally and in poultices, primarily as a vasoconstrictor for vein disorders (venous insufficiency) and as a diuretic to remove fluids from the body; for lower leg and ankle swelling, itching, cramping, and aching heaviness in legs, varicose veins, spider veins, vein weakness with dark dry skin, ulcerative sores, blood clots (phlebitis, thrombosis) including after surgery, hemorrhoids, dizziness standing up; reduces capillary fragility, prevents atherosclerosis; diuretic, increases urine flow and reduces water retention for cystitis; use for bladder and kidney stones, kidney and bladder infections, urethritis, nephritis, edema, dropsy, gout, rheumatism, menstrual difficulties, and PMS; also used as a poultice for sprains and broken and dislocated bones; internally and as a poultice for respiratory dis-eases with difficult breathing and chest congestion; jaundice, headaches; laxative, appetite stimulant, increases sweating to reduce and break fevers; in cosmetic creams to tighten and soothe skin, cellulite, stretch marks, wrinkles, and around eyes. *Diuretic, anti-inflammatory, vein constricting.* Rare side effects of nausea and upset stomach; may worsen high blood pressure and benign prostate dis-ease but listed as safe in pregnancy; no confirmed drug interactions but may interfere with high blood pressure drugs.

Butterbur • *(Petasites hybridis, Petasites vulgaris)*

Used in Europe since the Middle Ages; only use preparations marked PA-free (pyrrolizidine alkaloids removed), as these alkaloids are liver toxic and possibly carcinogenic; positive potential for migraine sufferers, reduces frequency and intensity of migraines and relief from pain during migraines, works for even severe migraine conditions, also for headaches and neuralgia; effective nondrug alternative for hay fever and allergic rhinitis (nasal congestion), colds, asthma, considered as effective as pseudoephedrine without the drowsiness side effect; internal and external smooth muscle relaxant and antispasmodic for muscle and skeletal pain, backache, stammering, cough, whooping cough, cramps, spasms; diuretic, water retention, cystitis; heart tonic; prevents ulcers, reduces fever by increasing perspiration; anti-inflammatory for internal and external infections; stress reducer, external use for skin wounds. *Antispasmodic, anti-inflammatory, antihistamine, diuretic, cardiac tonic.* Use PA-free (no pyrrolzidine alkaloids) only; mild possible side effects of burping or indigestion; not for use in pregnancy or breastfeeding, for small children, with severe kidney or liver dis-ease, or if allergic to ragweed; no known drug interactions.

34

Calendula • *(Calendula officinalis)*

Also called pot marigold; best known in many homeopathic salves and ointments but also used internally in tinctures and capsules; internal and external healer that soothes the skin, mucous membranes, and digestive tract; use as a salve for skin moisturizing and all skin disorders, cuts, wounds, acne, minor infections, inflammation, bruises, sunburn, burns, bleeding, insect bites, eczema, psoriasis, diaper rash, cradle cap, herpes sores, gum ulcers; offers skin burn protection in cancer radiation therapy; used in eardrops for ear infection pain; internally used for intestinal inflammation, indigestion, colitis, stomach ulcers, bowel ulcers, diverticulitis, yeast overrun in the bowel, liver and gallbladder dis-eases, hepatitis, jaundice; increases bile flow; promotes sweating to break fevers, used to "break out" pending childhood eruptive dis-eases; reduces pain, thought to prevent gangrene and tetanus; soothes digestive tract after surgery; regulates the menstrual cycle, relieves cramps, may reduce conception; uterine stimulant; inflammatory pelvic dis-ease, varicose veins; may help reduce blood pressure. *Antifungal, anti-inflammatory, stimulant, astringent, antiseptic, wound healer.* No known side effects; do not use in pregnancy or breastfeeding, or if allergic; may increase effects of sedative drugs.

California Poppy • *(Eschscholzia californica)*

California state flower, also called golden poppy, distantly related to opium poppy but without opiate or narcotic constituents, nonaddictive; can be smoked for a legal euphoric sedative high (but a cup of the tea is stronger); calms the nerves, acts as a sedative, promotes sleep without grogginess the next morning; can be used for overexcited children who won't go to sleep, nervous tension, anxiety, agitation, hyperactivity; pain relief especially for pain with anxiety; inflammatory or arthritis pain, colic, toothache, coughs; relieves constipation and bedwetting; internal and external cleanser and detoxifier; cleanses the gallbladder, increases cellular nutrient absorption, oxygenates the circulatory system, helps in the assimilation of vitamin A. *Antispasmodic, sedative, analgesic.* Often combined with other herbs for sleep or calming; no side effects or aftereffects; not for use with sleeping pills, not recommended in pregnancy or breastfeeding, or for children under six years.

Cascara Sagrada • *(Rhamnus purshiana)*

Standard herb for treating constipation; can be used alone but is more often combined with senna and other herbs; laxative, colon cleanser and toner; stimulates peristaltic action of the large intestine, expels worms and parasites, used for acute and chronic constipation, prevents constipation from becoming chronic, prevents laxative dependency by promoting regularity, not habit forming, doesn't deplete the body of nutrients; reduces the length of illnesses by cleaning toxins from the body, eliminates cancer cells and bacterial toxins from the digestive tract and body, thus preventing colon cancer and inflammatory bowel dis-eases (diverticulitis, Crohn's dis-ease, colitis, ileitis, irritable bowel syndrome), promotes balance of beneficial bacteria in the intestines, reduces yeast overruns; stimulates the entire gastrointestinal tract, stomach, liver, gallbladder, pancreas, colon; promotes normal gastric secretions, increases bile flow, opens bile ducts, prevents and clears gallstones, indigestion, gas, jaundice, liver congestion, liver dis-eases, increases appetite, reduces obesity; also regulates the pituitary gland and balances endocrine system, calms, aids insomnia; may be immunosuppressant for use in skin grafts, leukemia, and autoimmune disorders. *Laxative, anti-spasmodic, antibacterial, liver stimulant, bitter tonic.* Possible side effects include cramps, nausea, irritation of intestines, dehydration, electrolyte imbalance; not for use in pregnancy, nursing, for small children, or if appendicitis is possible; use with expert advice with chronic diarrhea, ulcers, inflammatory bowel dis-eases, heart dis-ease, hernia, severe anemia, kidney or liver dis-ease; may interact with digitalis.

Castor Oil • *(Ricinus communis)*
Palma christi, Edgar Cayce's favorite remedy, the greatest all-healer; use externally in castor oil warm packs, compresses, or as a salve; use internally only as a laxative (adults, 1 to 4 tablespoons; children two to twelve years, 1 to 3 teaspoons); primary use is external for uterine fibroids, menstrual difficulties, endometriosis, mastitis, breast irritations especially from nursing, lumpy cystic breasts; increases breast milk, prevents miscarriage, brings on labor at end of pregnancy; for abdominal discomfort of all kinds, appendicitis (external use only, never as a laxative if appendicitis is suspected), liver and gallbladder dis-eases, hepatitis, immune function,

sciatica and back pain, intestinal dis-eases and obstructions, infections, sores, abscesses, headaches and migraines, inflammations of all kinds, cancer, eye irritations, earaches and ear infections, children's hyperactivity. *Antitoxic, antiviral, antifungal, antibacterial, anticancer, laxative.* Internal use warning: never take laxatives with abdominal pain, nausea, vomiting, or possibility of appendicitis, may be habit forming; easier-to-take laxatives are available; no known side effects or drug interactions with external use. To make a castor oil pack (best used at bedtime), wet a washcloth or other absorbent cloth with castor oil. Place it on the area of the body to be treated. Cover with plastic wrap to keep it in place and to keep in the messiness, then put a towel over it. Place a warm but not uncomfortably hot heating pad over the area for an hour to an hour and a half, then leave the pack on for the rest of the night. Repeat nightly if needed. Clean oil off of skin in the morning with baking soda and water. Keep the same pack in a plastic container to reuse.

Catnip • *(Nepeta cataria)*

About two-thirds of cats are susceptible to this cat aphrodisiac; it is a no-harm high but should not be given to diabetic cats or overexcitable cats with heart dis-ease; in essential oil form, catnip is a mosquito repellent ten times stronger than DEET; planted in the garden it repels insects from other plants; human use in capsules, tea, or tinctures; diarrhea (best-choice remedy), upset stomach, gas, nausea, hiccups, stomach cramps, acid stomach, indigestion, colic in babies (as a diluted tea with chamomile); mild sedative for insomnia, prevents nightmares, reduces restlessness and nervousness, antispasmodic; brings on menses and increases menstrual flow, aids menstrual cramps and PMS, heals morning sickness, prevents miscarriage and premature birth; use as a poultice for sore breasts when nursing; aids muscle cramps; use topically for skin sores and hemorrhoids; use strained, cooled tea in a hair rinse for dandruff; promotes sweating for use in breaking up colds, flu, fevers, and childhood infectious dis-eases; soothes nervous system and digestive system; use in a poultice or compress for tonsillitis and toothache; chew for toothache and headaches; catnip can be smoked as a legal substitute for marijuana, causing euphoria and visual hallucinations in people. *Antispasmodic, increases sweating, antigas, tonic, sedative, astringent.* Very safe when used in normal dosage; possible minor overdose effects include fatigue, nausea, vomiting, headache, or skin allergy; caution in pregnancy, breastfeeding; use diluted for infants; not for those with pelvic inflammatory dis-ease, or those taking sleeping pills or antidepressant drugs.

Cat's Claw • *(Uncaria tormentosa)*

Also called una de gato (Spanish for "claw of the cat"), and known as the "sacred herb" of the South American rain forest; works to prevent and treat dis-ease and to normalize the body's functions, especially used for immune system dis-eases, HIV, and cancer; prevents RNA mutation (antimutagenic), stops production and development of cancer cells and viral replication in AIDS, may dissolve cancer cells, retards tumor growth, reduces side effects in AIDS and cancer treatment (drug, radiation, and chemotherapy damage), prevents opportunistic infections in cancer and AIDS patients; can be used along with medical therapies and drugs; shows promise in most types of cancer, including brain tumors, breast cancer, leukemia, melanoma, cervical cancer, prostate cancer, and more; also used for all infections and inflammations (fever, viruses, sinus, colds, flu, sore throat, earaches, eye infections); gastrointestinal and respiratory dis-eases (ulcers, gastritis, asthma, indigestion); joint dis-ease (arthritis, rheumatism, bursitis, bone pain, backache, tendonitis, stiffness and swelling); immune disorders (chronic fatigue, environmental illness, toxic exposure, fibromyalgia, allergies); intestinal inflammatory dis-eases (Crohn's dis-ease, colitis, diverticulitis, diarrhea, dysentery, hemorrhoids); expels parasites and worms, lowers blood pressure and cholesterol, normalizes blood sugar (diabetes, hypoglycemia); skin dis-eases (acne, deep wounds, warts, psoriasis, herpes, shingles, athlete's foot); Alzheimer's, multiple sclerosis, and other central nervous system dis-eases; menstrual cycle regulator; stops uterine hemorrhage, aids recovery after childbirth, use for urinary tract infections and PMS; may be contraceptive; also used for stress, depression, general pain, debility, and more; blood purifier, kidney cleanser. *Antioxidant, antimutagenic, anticancer, antiviral, anti-inflammatory, cell protector.* Works well with most medical drugs and with MSM (methylsulfonylmethane, a dietary supplement), pau d'arco, medicinal mushrooms, Essiac, and other herbs; mild side effects of diarrhea or constipation; some sources say not for autoimmune dis-eases, multiple sclerosis, or tuberculosis, not in pregnancy or breastfeeding; avoid with hormonal drugs, insulin, and vaccines.

Cayenne Pepper • *(Capsicum)*

Hot spice and remedy that works by heating to increase circulation and acts as a counterirritant; increases the power of other herbs and supplements; use internally in capsules or externally in a cream, also as a cooking spice (red pepper); stimulates all secreting organs, aids digestion when taken with meals or used as a food spice, aids weight loss, diabetes (regulates blood sugar levels), antioxidant, reduces fevers, chills; laxative, appetite stimulant, decongestant; reduces internal tumors, antioxidant and decongestant for colds (with honey); use externally for arthritis, muscle pain, shingles (after blisters disappear), nerve pain of all kinds, fibromyalgia, post-surgical pain, pain after amputation, pain from peripheral neuropathy from diabetes (but not from HIV), back pain, psoriasis, sore throat (gargle), as a nasal for cluster migraines (expert advice needed); promising remedy for heart dis-ease from atherosclerotic (clogged) arteries; increases circulation, aids circulatory disorders, and helps normalize irregular heart rhythm. *Stimulant, antioxidant, rubefacient, antiseptic, tonic, circulatory stimulant, digestive.* When using external creams, pain may increase at first then greatly lessens; may cause skin irritation, remove from skin with vinegar; avoid getting in eyes, wash hands after using; do not use after hot showers or with a heating pad; may cause stomach irritation; the burning sensations are uncomfortable but cause no harm; use as a cooking spice but not in medical doses while pregnant or nursing; many drug interactions, research your medication before using.

Celery Seed • *(Apium graveolens)*
Garden celery; primarily used as a diuretic for joint and kidney dis-eases, tones and purifies blood and kidneys, supports heart health; promotes urine flow and release of uric acid and toxins from the kidneys; antiseptic to reduce inflammation; relieves joint pain, arthritis, rheumatism, gout, neuralgia, cystitis, nephritis, kidney congestion, water retention,

bloating, promotes weight loss; digestive bitter for indigestion, poor digestion, hiccups, gas, appetite stimulant, laxative (high in fiber); spleen support, liver stimulant; reduces jaundice, reduces incidence of colorectal cancer, protects the liver from aspirin and ibuprofen side effects and damage; relaxes the blood vessels (vasodilator), reduces high blood pressure and high cholesterol, stabilizes heart rate, reduces palpitations and angina, lessens heart workload by clearing excess fluids, and reduces blood sugar levels—all primarily because of its diuretic action; brings on menses, relieves PMS, contracts the uterus, stops bleeding, aids in recovery after childbirth, increases breast milk; also for bronchitis, colds, flu, prevents tumor formation; relaxant, reduces muscle spasms, calms the nerves, promotes sleep. *Diuretic, antiseptic, antiinflammatory, sedative, antirheumatic, antigas.* Possible side effects of diarrhea, indigestion, increased photosensitivity, allergy; avoid overdosing and overuse, avoid in pregnancy, with kidney dis-ease or infection, or if taking blood thinners or diuretic drugs; buy celery seed from a health food or herbal source, because garden seeds are treated with fungicides and insecticides.

Chamomile • *(Matricaria recutita)*

The best all-round herbal for babies and children, and safe in pregnancy, nursing, and for long-term use; easily available in tea bags at any supermarket; good for adults too; use for nervousness, emotional upset, restlessness, anxiety, insomnia, colic and teething pain in babies, nausea, earache, asthma, fevers, childhood infectious dis-eases, intestinal worms, flu symptoms, and diarrhea, especially in children; prevents nightmares; cleans and heals wounds and ulcers (of all kinds, internally and externally); burns, including those from radiation therapy, inflamed skin and mucous membranes, skin irritations of all kinds, eczema, mouth and gum dis-ease; diuretic for cystitis and kidney infections, appetite tonic; aids PMS, brings on menses; use for headaches, indigestion, heartburn, gas, upper respiratory irritation (*see* Eyebright for eye irritation), stomach ulcers, ulcers and irritation of entire gastrointestinal tract, inflammation and inflammatory dis-eases, allergic reactions, hangovers; good as a lightening hair rinse for blondes, as a sitz bath or salve for hemorrhoids, in baths for muscle aches and fatigue, in salve for wounds and skin irritations, in compresses for neuralgia and toothache, in tea for emotional stress; use as a weak tea with peppermint or catnip for babies' colic. *Anti-inflammatory, antispasmodic, analgesic, calmative, antifungal, antiallergenic, diuretic, tonic, digestive.* Although rare, people allergic to ragweed may be allergic to chamomile; possible interactions with blood thinners and other drugs—research your medication.

Chaparral Leaf • *(Larrea tridentata, Larrea species)*
Inhibits several inflammation-causing enzymes, is an antihistamine, antiprostaglandin, fights fungus, and inhibits tumor growth, but may not be safe because of liver toxicity; use for inflammatory conditions, allergic reactions, respiratory infections, sinus congestion, asthma, cramps, irregular menses, diarrhea, *Candida albicans*, colds, flu, sore throat, urinary tract infections; helps in stopping smoking; anticancer and antitumor properties may reduce uterine fibroids, cystic breasts, and internal and external benign and cancerous tumors; use externally for skin dis-eases and parasites, eczema, ringworm, skin fungus, herpes, athlete's foot (can be combined with tea tree oil), chicken pox sores, snakebites, cold sores, wounds; use as a poultice for joint pain, arthritis,

rheumatism, sciatic and back pain, neuritis (nerve) pain. *Antibacterial, antiamoebic, antioxidant, anticancer, antiseptic, anti-inflammatory, antiprostaglandin, antimicrobial, diuretic, tonic.* Do not overdose or overuse; use other safer herbs wherever possible; stop if symptoms of nausea, fever, fatigue, jaundice, or dark-colored urine occur; do not use if you have liver dis-ease; not for use in pregnancy or breastfeeding.

Chaste Tree Berry • *(Vitex agnus-castus)*

Also known as vitex; used almost exclusively for normalizing and regulating women's hormones and cycles; normalizes estrogen-to-progesterone balance; an adaptogen possibly affecting the pituitary and hypothalamus rather than the reproductive hormones directly; used for PMS for symptoms of bloating, cramps, hormonal headaches, hormonal constipation, anxiety, irritability, mood swings, water retention, hormonal acne, breast tenderness, painful periods, lack of periods (amenorrhea), irregular periods; restores normal cycles after stopping use of oral contraceptives, promotes fertility, may help prevent miscarriage, increases breast milk after childbirth (higher doses decrease breast milk); also used for endometriosis, fibrocystic breast dis-ease, fibroid tumors, and uterine inflammation; a safe alternative to hormone replacement therapy for menopause and postmenopausal symptoms; stops irregular perimenopausal bleeding, heavy menstrual bleeding, increases duration of sleep, antitumor; in men, reduces overactive libido, adult acne, benign prostate enlargement; may prevent prostate cancer; reproductive system tonic; takes two to three months for full therapeutic effects; side effects include skin rash, itching, nausea, dry mouth, headaches, increased menstrual bleeding (rare) or between-period bleeding, fast heartbeat, hair loss; use in pregnancy and breastfeeding only with expert advice; not recommended with hormone-sensitive cancers or conditions, hormone replacement therapy, or oral contraceptives; avoid with Parkinson's dis-ease or schizophrenia.

Cherry Juice • *(Prunus cerasus)*

This is tart cherry juice, not the sweet cherries from the supermarket; must be taken raw, can be bought in juice, juice concentrate, or in capsules; diabetics look for sugar-free formulas; contains high levels of vitamin C, superoxide dismutase (SOD), potassium, melatonin, flavinoids, and anthrocyanins; clears uric acid from the body and prevents crystal buildup in the joints; an anti-inflammatory more powerful than aspirin that inhibits the COX-1 and COX-2 enzymes implicated in joint dis-ease without the side effects of aspirin or NSAIDS; brings almost miraculous pain relief and increase in joint mobility to sufferers of gout, rheumatoid arthritis, osteoarthritis, and all joint dis-eases; prevents joint damage; also effective for heel spurs, tendonitis, muscle fatigue, lupus, post-polio syndrome, connective tissue dis-eases and injuries, fibromyalgia, spinal disk dis-ease, back pain, neck pain, carpal tunnel syndrome, Sjogren's syndrome, insomnia, headaches; reduces muscle pain, fatigue, and loss of strength after hard exercise; prevents and treats kidney dis-ease, kidney stones, cystitis, indigestion, stomach ulcers, constipation, irritable bowel syndrome, anemia; aids in weight loss (good with apple juice); lowers cholesterol, protects artery walls from plaque buildup and damage; prevents heart dis-ease and stroke, blood clots, cancer, varicose veins (strengthens vein walls), cataracts; slows aging. *Anti-inflammatory, antioxidant, diuretic.* There are many testimonials of pain reduction and healing of many dis-eases

A
B
C
D
E
F
G
H
I
J
K
L
M
N
O
P
Q
R
S
T
U
V
W
X
Y
Z

with tart cherry juice; possible diarrhea side effect; no known warnings or drug interactions.

Chickweed • *(Stellaria media)*

Pervasive weed with high nutritional content, rich in vitamin C, a tasty salad green, also use steamed and in soups; use to cool hot conditions, moisturize dryness, and draw out toxins; external skin uses include rashes, infections, inflammations, ulcers, boils, carbuncles, abscesses, diaper rash, psoriasis, swelling, eczema, sores, scabs, itching, insect bites; dissolves warts and cysts; used in many skin-care preparations; used as an external poultice over the abdomen to cool the liver; also used as poultice for muscles cramps, tendonitis, rheumatism, hemorrhoids, earache; poultice and eyewash for inflamed eyes and conjunctivitis; internal use for lung congestion, bronchitis, coughs, hoarseness, asthma, whooping cough, expectorant; aids digestion and absorption of nutrients, balances intestinal flora, yeast overrun; bowel detoxifier; used for constipation, obesity, stomach ulcers, anemia; hormone balancer, douche for trichomonal vaginal infection, PMS; diuretic, water retention, cystitis, arthritis; liver tonic, reduces effects of alcohol abuse on the liver. *Tonic, diuretic, expectorant, coolant, antioxidant, blood cleanser, wound healer.* Extreme overuse can theoretically cause nitrate poisoning (weakness, headache, fainting, dizziness); should not be used internally in pregnancy, while nursing, or for infants; no known drug interactions.

Chlorella • *(Chlorella vulgaris, Chlorella pyrenoidosa)*
Highly nutritious single-celled green algae, called a green food; takes three to six months of use for full effects to become evident; detoxifies the body and all its organs and functions, binds with toxins to remove them from the body through the bowels, promotes healthy acid-alkaline balance, increases beneficial flora in the intestines, increases energy and iron levels; removes pesticides, chemicals, radiation, heavy metals, and pollutants from the body, reduces cellular damage, promotes optimal function of all organs and systems, cleanses the blood; immune enhancer, antitumor and anticancer; increases resistance to viruses and bacteria, protects from chemotherapy and radiation treatment damage, improves digestion and assimilation, protects mucous membranes of the gastrointestinal tract; lowers cholesterol, balances high or low blood pressure, lowers

triglycerides, prevents blood clots, prevents damage to the cardiovascular system, reduces heart attacks and strokes, promotes heart function; normalizes high or low blood sugar levels (diabetes and hypoglycemia); use for all immune and degenerative dis-eases, cancer, AIDS, Epstein-Barr, chronic fatigue, fibromyalgia, chronic viral dis-eases, respiratory viruses and colds; liver dis-ease and damage, kidney dis-ease, digestive disorders, anemia, bad breath, constipation, peptic ulcers, skin dis-eases and wounds, brain and mental function, aging. *Adaptogen, anticancer, immune booster, detoxifier, antioxidant.* Detoxification die-off symptoms may occur soon after beginning use and last for a short time: diarrhea, constipation, lethargy, fatigue, nausea, photosensitivity, irritability; a few people are allergic (indicated by burping up the taste of chlorella or by hives); safe for children but not recommended for pregnant or breastfeeding women; not for use by those on blood-thinning medications.

Cilantro Extract • *(Coriandrum sativum)*
This is the leaf extract of the culinary spice coriander, also called Chinese parsley; compare prices, some brands are more expensive than others; removes heavy metals (lead,

mercury, aluminum) from the body, detoxifies so that formerly resistant infections can be healed, including herpes simplex 1 and 2, CMV (cytomegalovirus), *Chlamydia trachomatis*; potential for cancer and HIV treatment; used with other herbs (alfalfa, nettles, chlorella) as an organ protector and to aid elimination; antifungal and antibacterial that also inactivates *E. coli*, *Salmonella*, and *Streptococcus* dis-ease organisms that result in fat rancidity and food poisoning; stomach soother for indigestion, gas, diarrhea, cramps, colic in infants, diarrhea; liver protector; disguises taste of less palatable herbs in some herbal combinations; other uses: anxiety, insomnia, headache, conjunctivitis, mouth ulcers, arthritis inflammation, aphrodisiac; external use for cuts, scrapes, infected wounds, and swellings. *Antioxidant, antibacterial, antifungal, anti-inflammatory, stimulant, detoxifier, digestive.* Should not be used for heavy metal detoxification programs if you have silver amalgam dental fillings; otherwise no restrictions unless allergic to coriander/cilantro; no known drug interactions.

54

Cinnamon Bark • *(Cinnamomum verum)*

A half teaspoon of common cinnamon per day can decrease blood sugar, blood pressure, cholesterol, and triglyceride levels by 20 percent in noninsulin diabetics; mix with oatmeal, also available in capsules; remedy for diarrhea, kills bacteria that causes cystitis, botulism, and food poisoning; also kills *Candida albicans* (yeast overrun), aflatoxin (a carcinogen) from fungus and mold, and other fungal, bacterial, and viral infections; expels worms and parasites; helps with weight loss, loss of appetite, fever, chills, flu, colds, cough with mucus, indigestion, nausea, vomiting, abdominal and chest pain, kidney dis-ease, bad breath, and toothache (in mouthwash); increases circulation in the extremities (feet, toes, fingers), whole body circulation for backache, muscle aches, impotence, and overall weakness; immune booster; relaxant, reduces anxiety and stress, warms; in women, reduces breast milk, stops uterine hemorrhage, cramps, menopausal pain and bleeding; external poultices for arthritis, rheumatism, toothache, headache, muscle pain, neuralgia, wounds, and athlete's foot. *Antimicrobial, antiviral, antioxidant, antibacterial, antifungal, analgesic, astringent, stimulant, digestive tonic.* Rare allergy and overdose symptoms include hot flushed skin, dizziness, rapid breathing, rapid pulse, shortness of breath, sweating, excitement and then drowsiness, inflamed gums, inflamed mouth and tongue, cracked lips, too low blood sugar; should not be used in pregnancy except as a food spice; seek expert advice with diabetes and prostate dis-ease; not for use with blood thinners, may inactivate antibiotics.

Coleus • *(Coleus forskohlii)*

Member of the mint family, active ingredient has been named forskolin; support for congestive heart failure; promotes healthy heart contractions, reduces angina and high blood pressure, prevents blood clots; vasodilator (widens blood vessels to increase blood flow), stroke preventive, after-stroke recovery, cerebral vascular insufficiency; decreases histamine release to reduce allergies and allergic reactions; bronchodilator used for asthma, bronchitis, hay fever; reduces inner-eye pressure from glaucoma; balances thyroid function; stops spasms of menstrual cramps, colic, irritable bowel syndrome; prevents cancer from metastasizing; also use for urinary infections, painful urination, obesity, insomnia, convulsions, skin rashes, eczema, and psoriasis. *Vasodilator, antihistamine, anti-spasmodic, anti-inflammatory.* No listed side effects but avoid getting in the eyes; caution in pregnancy and nursing; may increase stomach acid, do not use with stomach ulcers; avoid with blood thinners, including aspirin, and with high blood pressure medications.

Coltsfoot • *(Tussilago farfara)*

Pervasive weed used medicinally since prehistory for coughs and respiratory dis-eases; can be smoked to draw the herb into the lungs, or used as tea, tincture, or capsules; primary use is as a suppressant for dry, irritating coughs and sore throats from all sources; expectorant (mucus thinner); respiratory congestion, wheezing, shortness of breath, whooping cough, flu, smoker's cough, lung ailments, bronchitis, laryngitis, emphysema, silicosis, mouth irritation, asthma; used in many commercial cough syrups and remedies; soothes digestion, stomach and intestines; diuretic; antidiarrhea; may have positive effect on beneficial bacteria in the intestines and reduces harmful bacteria; use externally for skin disorders and irritations, eczema, ulcers, wounds, rashes, sores, joint pain;

immune stimulant that may help increase immune resistance to dis-ease. *Antispasmodic, anti-inflammatory, expectorant, soothing, diuretic, tonic.* Often used with licorice root or wild cherry bark; generally considered safe with normal dosage and short-term use, no side effects but potentially liver toxic when overdosed or used long term; not for use by infants or during pregnancy (may be abortifacient); not for use with some high blood pressure drugs.

Comfrey • *(Symphytum officinale)*
Women have used this herb for thousands of years, but today's information suggests a warning of liver failure or even cancer with internal overuse; most use today is by compresses and poultices applied externally; speeds natural replacement of body cells, reduces swelling and inflammation, reduces bruising, stops bleeding, heals damaged and injured tissues, heals bones, prevents and reduces scarring; use for broken bones, sprains, wounds, arthritis, varicose-vein ulcers, diabetic leg and foot ulcers, gangrene conditions, acne and skin discomfort of all kinds, burns, and diaper rash; wet a fresh raw leaf in hot water and place it on skin wound or rash for instant soothing and

healing; use the tincture with goldenseal (one-third goldenseal, two-thirds comfrey in a spray bottle) as a highly effective all-healer of skin infections, sores, burns, and wounds for people and animals; traditionally used internally for bronchial and lung dis-eases, diarrhea, dysentery, sore throats (gargle), mouth sores (rinse), whooping cough, tuberculosis, internal hemor-rhages (use tea or tincture of witch hazel herb instead), and gas-tric ulcers, and to decrease menstrual flow; use strained, cooled tea in a hair rinse with nettles for soft, shining hair; use as a sitz bath or salve for vaginal dryness and itching in menopausal women; use as tea; use whole leaves in the garden as fertilizer and mulch, and in making compost; it is highly nutritional for all plants. *Anti-inflammatory, astringent, expectorant, lubricant, analgesic, wound healer.* Caution with internal use, the medical system says it is liver toxic, best used externally; no known side effects or drug interactions with external use.

Coriander • *See* Cilantro

Corn Silk • *(Zea mays)*
Plant originating in the New World and known by Native

Americans for more than seven thousand years, the botanic name translates to "mother of life"; corn silk is the silky tassel inside the corn husk; primary use is as a diuretic without potassium loss mainly for urinary tract inflammation and infections, chronic and acute in women and men; soothes and tones the urinary tract, treats cystitis, urinary retention, urinary frequency, urethritis, blood in the urine, painful urination, urinary and kidney stones, urinary gravel, kidney infections and dis-eases, benign prostate dis-ease symptoms, swollen prostate; helps incontinence in elders and bedwetting in children; reduces frequency of chronic bladder and kidney infections, aids obesity due to water retention; use as a diuretic for high blood pressure; cardiac mild stimulant, heart dis-ease edema; lowers heart dis-ease risk; diabetes, lowers blood sugar; reduces blood-clotting time, stops bleeding, high in vitamin K; for PMS, bloating and water retention before menses, brings on menses, reduces menstrual pain; cleanses and detoxifies liver, promotes bile flow, prevents and heals liver dis-eases, gout, jaundice, malaria, hepatitis, cirrhosis; prevents gallstones; also for carpal tunnel syndrome, mumps, gonorrhea, asthma, boils, arthritis. *Diuretic, anti-inflammatory, antispasmodic, antiseptic,*

A
B
C
D
E
F
G
H
I
J
K
L
M
N
O
P
Q
R
S
T
U
V
W
X
Y
Z

analgesic, antiviral, lubricant, tonic. Safe with normal use; may cause dehydration in children; side effects: possible allergic reaction or low potassium with overuse; may interact with warfarin and some diabetic and antihypoglycemia drugs.

Cramp Bark • *(Viburnum opulus)*

Used interchangeably with black haw herb (*Viburnum prunifolium*); relaxes muscles by blocking the enzyme that causes spasms; useful for every muscle in the body (internal and external), every discomfort resulting from muscle spasms and overcontraction, and every pain associated with movement; use for muscle pain and tension, cramps of all kinds (menstrual, uterine, muscle cramps, stomach or intestinal cramps), irritable bowel syndrome, constipation, headaches, contracted muscles in arthritis, joint pain, back pain, pain of mumps and swollen glands, lockjaw; also use for menstrual and menopausal pain and blood loss, brings on delayed or too light menses, treats threatened miscarriage, hormonal migraines, and endometriosis; sedative, calms and soothes the nerves, nervous tension, nervous disorders, seizures; lowers blood pressure, heart palpitations; improves blood circulation, circulatory dis-eases, heart dis-ease; rheumatism, breathing difficulties, asthma, colic. *Antispasmodic, anti-inflammatory, sedative, astringent.* Little research has been done on this herb, no known side effects, warnings, or drug interactions.

Cranberry • *(Vaccinium macrocarpon)*
Available in juice or capsules, tinctures are very high in alcohol and less effective; supermarket cranberry juice contains a high amount of sugar that can be avoided by using health food store concentrates, but concentrates without sugar are very sour and unpleasant tasting; supermarket juices are effective and are safe if you are not diabetic; capsules are less effective than juices, but they can be found sugar-free and they work; to stop a urinary tract infection with cranberry juice, drink one large glassful every hour until symptoms stop; to prevent urinary infections, drink one large glassful per day; for capsules, tinctures, and concentrates, follow label for dosage; best possible remedy for cystitis, urinary tract and kidney infections, urinary gravel, kidney stones, bleeding cystitis, strong-smelling urine; works by preventing *E. coli* bacteria (and other bacteria) from sticking to the

walls of the bladder and urethra, and probably by acidifying the urine (that it acidifies is under dispute); after receiving dozens of yellow jacket wasp stings and waking up very sick from them, a glass of cranberry juice seemed to neutralize the venom, and very quickly; other uses: can neutralize *H. pylori* bacteria that causes stomach ulcers and dental plaque (more effective if oregano oil is added to the cranberry juice), and may do the same for cancer cells; antioxidant that may help prevent heart dis-ease, relax blood vessels, lower cholesterol, and prevent cholesterol from sticking to artery walls; may increase vitamin B_{12} absorption, stimulate brain function, enhance memory, treat anorexia nervosa, increase speed of wound healing, dissolve gallstones, stimulate stomach and liver function, and prevent stomach and liver dis-ease. *Antioxidant, anticancer, antibacterial, antiseptic.* Extremely safe, including in pregnancy, with diarrhea and indigestion the only side effects; diabetics need sugar-free formulations; cranberry may counteract antacids, may increase excretion of some drugs, can theoretically (but not likely) increase the effectiveness of blood thinners and cause bleeding.

Damiana • *(Turnera diffusa, Turnera aphrodisiaca)*

Widely touted as an aphrodisiac and used in many sexual enhancement combination formulas for men and women; balances deficiencies but has no overstimulating effect on normal function; euphoric similar to the effects of marijuana; mimics the action of progesterone and may be useful for progesterone deficiency (usually in menopause), is not estrogenic (does not stimulate estrogen or estrogen-receptive cancers or conditions); balances and tones the glandular and hormonal systems, central nervous system, and digestive system; relieves depression, stress, nervous tension, mental chatter, nervous debility, exhaustion, weakness, mood disorders, headaches, anxiety, hypochondria, dizziness, poor physical balance, bedwetting; may be useful for paralytic dis-eases, including Lou Gehrig's dis-ease and Parkinson's dis-ease; lowers blood sugar, relieves internal and external muscular spasms; digestive stimulant (bitter); use for indigestion, laxative, colic, ulcers, dysentery, appetite suppressant, aid to weight loss; expectorant (thins and expels mucus), cough suppressant; use for colds, flu, lung congestion, viral infections, earaches, eye inflammation, asthma, bronchitis, emphysema; tones the reproductive system, increases libido in men and women, stimulates orgasm, aids impotence; aid for infertility, childbirth, sexually transmitted dis-eases; also regulates menstrual cycles, PMS, menopausal symptoms, hot flashes, menstrual headaches, relieves vaginal dryness, normalizes female hormone levels; traditional use as abortifacient. *Antispasmodic, antidepressant, astringent, bitter, expectorant, diuretic, tonic, hormone balancer, aphrodisiac.* Not for use in pregnancy, while breastfeeding, or for children; may reduce iron absorption, lowers blood sugar levels; no listed side effects or drug interactions.

Dandelion • *(Taraxacum officinale)*

Salad green and spring tonic herb that grows everywhere and is considered a nuisance on most northern lawns; can be used as a coffee substitute; place fresh leaves in a bag with unripe fruit to ripen the fruit quickly; primarily used as a liver cleanser and healer, and a diuretic that does not deplete potassium from the body; use for all liver dis-eases and congestion, jaundice, hepatitis, cirrhosis, gallbladder function; increases bile production, spleen function; reduces side effects of drugs processed by the liver; diuretic and blood purifier for kidneys, urinary tract, cystitis, urinary and kidney stones and gravel, water retention, edema from high blood pressure and heart weakness; lowers total cholesterol, increases good HDL cholesterol, lowers triglycerides, balances and lowers blood sugar (hypoglycemia and diabetes); also for anemia, nervousness, spring tonic, laxative, stomach irritation, indigestion, heartburn, appetite stimulant, rheumatism, and joint pain; may improve beneficial bacteria in intestines; plant sap dabbed on repeatedly dissolves warts; cosmetic lotions fade freckles and clear skin, inflammatory skin conditions, acne, and eczema. *Diuretic, tonic, stimulant, laxative.* Minor side effects may include skin allergy, stomach upset, heartburn, diarrhea; use with expert advice with liver or gallbladder dis-ease; may worsen lithium side effects and interact with diuretics, blood thinners, and diabetes medications.

Dill Weed • (*Anethum graveolens*)

Kitchen spice and flavoring for pickles, soups, vinegars, and many other foods; rich in calcium, minerals, and fiber; used for healing since Roman times and longer; major indigestion remedy and stomach soother for infants, children, and adults;

use for gas, colic, overeating, dyspepsia, hiccups, intestinal spasms and cramps, constipation, breath freshening; relaxes the muscles of the digestive tract; increases breast milk, can be given for infant indigestion through the breast milk when eaten by the nursing mother, promotes babies' sleep; also used for wound healing (powder of burned seeds used externally), coughs, colds, flu, headaches; reduces sweating; new research lists it as a chemo-protective food that can neutralize some carcinogens and pollutants (cigarette smoke, charcoal grill smoke, and smoke from burning trash); stops the overgrowth of bacteria, yeast, and mold; source of calcium to reduce bone loss and osteoporosis. *Stimulant, aromatic, stomach soothing, antispasmodic.* No known cautions or drug interactions, but can cause dermatitis and sun sensitivity in some people; high in salt content.

Dong Quai • *(Angelica sinesis)*
Women's ginseng, reproductive toner, and healer for long-term use; takes eight to twelve weeks for full effect; tastes like fresh celery or parsley; uterine tonic, estrogen balancer (contains no estrogenic properties itself), relaxes and contracts the uterus,

strengthens women's reproductive hormones and system, alternative to hormone replacement therapy drugs in menopause; helps regulate menstrual cycles; use for painful and abnormal menstruation (dysmenorrhea), lack of menstruation (amenorrhea), irregular menstrual bleeding, PMS, cramps, to restore cycles after taking birth control pills; aids childbirth and eases delivery, post-childbirth healing; use for hormonal acne and migraines, fibrocystic breast dis-ease, chronic pelvic disorders, polycystic ovaries, recovery from traumatic injury to reproductive organs, yeast overruns, and vaginal infections; use for all menopausal symptoms: vaginal dryness, irregular periods, night sweats, hot flashes, fibroid tumors, blood-loss anemia, hormonal migraines and headaches; also for ulcers, carbuncles, pain relief; increases urination; general muscle relaxant, laxative; use for shingles, insomnia, chronic nasal congestion, rheumatoid arthritis, allergies, respiratory tonic, infections; heart tonic and healer for heart arrhythmia, chest pain, increasing exercise tolerance, increased circulation; prevents atherosclerosis (arterial plaque), lowers blood pressure (pressure may rise temporarily first), reduces brain damage after strokes; liver healer and cleanser; use for hepatitis,

A
B
C
D
E
F
G
H
I
J
K
L
M
N
O
P
Q
R
S
T
U
V
W
X
Y
Z

Herb Listings

cirrhosis; enhances protein metabolism. *Analgesic, antibacterial, antispasmodic, diuretic and cardio-tonic.* May increase sun sensitivity, causing sunburn, skin rashes, and skin inflammations; do not take in pregnancy or while nursing; do not use with blood thinner drugs or herbs; do not use while taking hormones or birth control pills without expert supervision; do not use the oil form of this herb.

Echinacea • *(Echinacea angustifolia)*

Much overused herbal antibiotic/herbal penicillin with no side effects; however, overuse can cause resistance to its benefits and lessen effectiveness; take for several days after symptoms end or the dis-ease may return; use for colds, cough, flu, pneumonia, bronchitis, sore throat, fever, infections, chronic fatigue syndrome (antiviral), gas and indigestion, cystitis, vaginal yeast infections (in a douche), ear infections; reduces inflammation and body pain; immune booster, blood cleanser, tonic; use externally for athlete's foot, skin infections, acne, ringworm; sinus infections, hay fever, wounds that don't heal (internally and externally), boils, burns, ulcers, eczema, venomous snakebites, toothache; traditional for mumps, measles, smallpox, arthritis (anti-inflammatory); not for long-term chronic dis-eases, including AIDS, tuberculosis, multiple sclerosis, or lupus, but may help in opportunistic infections from these dis-eases; it is in dispute whether echinacea prevents or shortens colds. *Antibiotic, antibacterial, antifungal, antiviral, antiprotozoa, antimicrobial, anti-inflammatory.* Possible side effects: diarrhea, indigestion, nausea, rash, bitter taste, tingling in mouth; should not be used with steroids or liver-toxic prescription medications.

Elderberry • *(Sambucus nigra, Sambucus canadensis)*

Has differing uses for flowers, leaves, and berries; the information here is for berries except where otherwise noted; the uncooked fresh plant is poisonous and the berries should not be eaten raw; major research on this herb has come from Israel; best use is for reducing the severity and length of flu and flu symptoms, and can clear colds or flu in seventy-two hours; fever, flu, diarrhea, colds, chills, bronchitis, coughs, cold sores, sore throat; high in vitamin C, induces sweating to break fevers, expels phlegm; diuretic; also used for nerve disorders, back pain, rheumatism, asthma, colic, croup; tonic

Herb Listings

for the reproductive and glandular systems; reduces intestinal inflammation; syrup dose is 1 teaspoon to 1 tablespoon twice a day for children, 2 teaspoons to 2 tablespoons twice a day for adults; *flowers* used externally in skin washes, skin astringent; reduces the appearance of freckles, lightens and tones skin, heals sunburn, burns, cuts, swelling, tightens capillaries; traditional ingredient in cosmetics; use as a tea internally for hay fever, sinusitis, kidney infections, diuretic, weight loss; *leaves* used externally for skin tumors, bruises, sprains, wounds, frostbite, and injuries; use internally as a tincture with Saint-John's-wort and soapwort to inhibit flu and herpes; use alone as a tea or tincture, as a diuretic for urinary and kidney infections, dropsy, edema, and constipation. *Antiviral, antibiotic, antibacterial, detoxifier, diuretic, immune enhancer, antioxidant, anti-inflammatory.* Dizziness and stupor are possible negative reactions in some people; not for use in pregnancy; no known drug interactions.

Elecampane • *(Inula helenium)*

Use for chronic lung infections and respiratory dis-eases as an expectorant to stop coughing and to thin and expel mucus;

deactivates the coughing reflex, strengthens and warms the lungs; also has antiseptic, antiviral, and antibacterial action; for colds, hacking coughs, flu, bronchitis, pneumonia, whooping cough, asthma, chronic obstructive pulmonary dis-ease (COPD), emphysema, tuberculosis; also for congestive heart failure with angina and shortness of breath; clears chronic discharges anywhere in the body (vaginitis, urinary) and excess mucus from the gastrointestinal tract, heals indigestion with debility, stimulates bile flow, expels intestinal worms; use for hemorrhoids, liver dis-eases, and hepatitis; brings on menses, breaks fever by promoting sweating; diuretic for water retention, PMS, bloating, edema, and urinary tract and kidney infections; aids depression; use internally and externally (poultice or compress) for skin dis-eases, scabies, impetigo, itching skin, sciatica, and neuralgia. *Expectorant, diuretic, antiseptic, antiparasitic, antibacterial.* Avoid if allergic to inulin (the herb's active ingredient), ragweed, sunflowers, asters, or other daisy-family plants; side effects with overuse or overdose include vomiting, diarrhea, irritated mouth and intestinal tract, spasms, palpitations, paralysis; not for use in pregnancy or nursing, or by diabetics; no known drug interactions.

Essiac • *See* Sheep Sorrel

Eucalyptus Leaf • *(Eucalyptus globulus, Eucalyptus folium)*
This is the plant leaf, *not* the essential oil (which should *never* be taken internally), of the Australian gum tree; works by its strong menthol odor; common ingredient in many over-the-counter remedies for sore muscles, colds, and flu: chest rubs, cough drops, throat lozenges, toothpaste, gargles, mouthwash, steam-kettle herbs, salves, ointments, bath salts, sports liniments; leaves may be smoked as a lung decongestant and also used as a tea; decongestant and expectorant for respiratory viruses and mucus, cough, colds, flu, bronchitis, nasal congestion, fever, chronic and acute ear infections (eardrop), sinusitis, hay fever, whooping cough, pneumonia, asthma, emphysema; use in topical salves and liniments for muscle aches and pains, fungus, wound disinfecting, bad breath, and to revive someone who has fainted; lowers blood sugar and increases insulin production for diabetes treatment; digestive and urinary tract antiseptic. *Antibacterial, antiseptic, anti-inflammatory, expectorant, antiviral, antimicrobial, stimulant, aromatic.* **The oil is poisonous when ingested.**

Leaf side effects include nausea, vomiting, and diarrhea; do not overuse; not for use in pregnancy or breastfeeding or for internal use by children; children under six should not use the cough drops, though steam-kettle and chest-rub use for children is safe; not for those with kidney, liver, or gastrointestinal tract inflammation, or high blood pressure; listed drug interactions are contradictory; research your medications and read package labels for safety warnings.

Evening Primrose Oil • *(Oenothera biennis)*

Known best in oil form, usually taken in capsules (2 capsules three times per day); primary constituents in evening primrose oil are gamma-linolenic acid and omega-6 essential fatty acid; use internally and externally for all skin irritations and dis-eases, eczema, rosacea, psoriasis, wounds and bruises, skin sores and fatigue in AIDS patients; female reproductive hormone balancer for menopausal symptoms, hot flashes, osteoporosis; use for high blood pressure, high cholesterol; prevents blood clots, prevents strokes and heart attacks, may be anticancer; use for PMS, breast cysts, breast cancer, breast soreness (mastitis, menstrual soreness), infertility, preeclampsia (high blood pressure during pregnancy); prevents premature childbirth and postnatal depression; eases labor pain during childbirth; prevents and heals nerve damage of all kinds, including diabetic neuropathy and chemotherapy-induced nerve damage; also for rheumatoid arthritis, asthma, stomachaches, hemorrhoids, kidney stones, and bowel disorders, including colitis, Crohn's dis-ease, and irritable bowel syndrome; promising for chronic fatigue, multiple sclerosis, obesity, ADHD, schizophrenia, cystic fibrosis, hepatitis B, lupus, and alcohol withdrawal (also reduces hangovers). *Hormone balancer, anticancer, anti-inflammatory, antioxidant.* Side effects can include contact allergy, headache, and indigestion; avoid with seizure disorders, can stimulate seizures in susceptible people; do not use with antipsychotic drugs (seizure risk), blood thinners, or aspirin.

Eyebright • *(Euphrasia officinalis)*

Used since the Middle Ages primarily for treatment of the eyes and vision; also an herbal antibacterial related to chamomile and goldenseal but less potent; use internally and externally; make a tea of 1 teaspoon of herb to a cup of boiled water, use the strained cooled-to-body-temperature tea as an eyewash and drink the rest; eyebright tea bags—cooled to body temperature—can be used as an eye poultice; strengthens sight, aids weakness of the eyes, eyestrain, all eye irritations and swellings, sties, conjunctivitis, blepharitis (inflamed eyelids), redness, watery eyes, oversensitivity to light, aging eyes, and all eye discomforts; said to restore vision; often mixed with goldenseal for eyewashes; use three to four times a day; use also for upper respiratory system colds and infections, irritation of upper respiratory mucous membranes, bronchitis, coughs (can be smoked), sinusitis, nose, throat, esophagus, allergies, and hay fever; reduces mucus, tightens mucous membranes, reduces runny nose, aids headaches, strengthens memory and thinking ability; also use for herpes sores, running eczema sores, skin wounds. *Antibacterial, antioxidant, antimucus, anti-inflammatory, astringent.* Side effects include confusion, nausea, sweating, pressure in the eye, itchy eyes, tearing, light sensitivity, swollen eyelids, vision changes; some people who are allergic to ragweed may be allergic to eyebright; preparations for use in the eye should be made and kept as sterile as possible; not recommended after eye surgeries; no known drug interactions.

False Unicorn Root • *(Chamaelirium luteum)*

Also called helonias root; almost exclusively used as a toner and restorative for women's reproductive system and its functions; use to balance the reproductive hormones, strengthen the position of bladder and uterus in the body, prevent and heal prolapsed uterus and bladder, feeling of dragging heaviness in the pelvis; strengthens and protects the ovaries, stimulates ovarian hormones, increases fertility, restores fertility and cycles after coming off the Pill; regulates the menstrual cycle, PMS, irregular menses, painful menses, hormonal depression, and irritability; use for morning sickness in pregnancy, threatened miscarriage, or for women with past miscarriages; use as recovery tonic after childbirth; restores uterine tone; helpful for menopausal symptoms, hormone replacement after early hysterectomy, hot flashes, vaginal dryness, mood swings, fibroid tumors, vaginal infections, endometriosis, pelvic inflammatory dis-ease, urinary incontinence; also a diuretic for cystitis, toner for the liver and kidneys; expels worms, relieves coughs (chewed), heals indigestion, nausea, lack of appetite; use for male impotence and prostate dis-ease. *Uterine tonic, diuretic, emetic, menstrual healer.* May cause vomiting if overdosed or overused but considered safe; use in pregnancy with expert advice; no listed drug interactions.

Fennel • *(Foeniculum vulgare)*

Culinary herb used much like dill weed for indigestion and respiratory viruses; use for stomach upset, gastritis, abdominal pain, digestive assimilation, nausea, morning sickness, babies' cramps, gas, colic, bloating, hiccups, breath freshener; laxative, prevents cramping with other laxatives; reduces hunger, promotes weight loss; opens blockages in liver, spleen, and gallbladder; increases flow of bile; use for jaundice, gout, hernia; blood cleanser; neutralizes toxins and poisons, snakebite; use for respiratory and minor viral dis-eases, including fever, chills, colds, croup, asthma, bronchitis, chronic coughs, wheezing, shortness of breath; expectorant, thins mucus, used in many cough syrups; tonic, aids recovery after illness; used as a wash for eye irritations and eyestrain; mild sedative, promotes sleep; improves the taste of other medicines; increases breast milk, has been used for breast enhancement, brings on menses; mild diuretic for urinary infections and kidney stones. *Antispasmodic,*

antimicrobial, antigas, weak diuretic, expectorant, mild stimulant.
Safe in normal doses; overdose can cause muscle cramps and
hallucinations; avoid with ciprofloxacin.

Fenugreek • *(Trigonella foenum-graecum)*
Food spice with a maple-syrup flavor, can also be eaten in
salads; the major ingredient in Lydia C. Pinkham's Vegetable
Compound for "female troubles"; major use is for increasing
breast milk production, usually within twenty-four to seventy-
two hours of starting treatment; can be discontinued when
enough lactation is achieved as long as the breasts are emp-
tied every few hours; protects against breast cancer; reduces
menstrual pain, menopause vaginal dryness; may enhance
breast size; male aphrodisiac, male libido; also for respiratory
infections and lung congestion, sinus, asthma, coughs, colds,
flu, bronchitis, sore throat, swollen glands, fever; expectorant
(loosens mucus), soothes; removes allergens and toxins from
the respiratory tract; immune stimulant, digestive aid; use for
colic, gas, diabetes, hyperthyroidism; lowers cholesterol, lowers triglycerides, lowers blood sugar; soothes peptic ulcers,
protects the liver from alcohol; use externally for wounds

and skin infections, dermatitis, eczema, chapped lips, boils, cysts, abscesses, burns. *Expectorant, soothes, stimulates breast milk, tonic, immune enhancer.* Side effects can include maple-smelling urine, nausea, sweating, dizziness, gas, diarrhea; can worsen asthma symptoms (difficulty breathing, fainting, hay fever type reactions); should not used in pregnancy, causes uterine contractions that may cause miscarriage; may increase bleeding risk in surgery; probable interactions with diabetes drugs, blood thinners, NSAIDS, and more—do the research if taking medical drugs.

Feverfew • (Tanacetum parthenium)

A promising nondrug hope for migraine sufferers when taken long term, use two or three fresh leaves brewed in a tea daily, or 60 to 120 drops of tincture twice a day, or 100 to 300 mg in capsule form up to four times a day; takes four to six weeks to take effect; reduces incidence of migraine up to 50 percent, prevents blood vessel spasms, contracts blood vessels; especially effective when taken with magnesium and vitamin B_2 (use full B complex); also use like aspirin but may be more effective than aspirin for rheumatoid arthritis, any chronic inflammation or inflammatory dis-ease; aids dizziness, tinnitus, nervous upset, hysteria, depression, headaches; improves digestion, expels intestinal worms, reduces fever; brings on menses, increases flow for sluggish menses, eases menstrual cramps; lowers blood pressure; blood thinner, appetite stimulant; acts as a tonic, causes sweating; use with honey for coughs, wheezing, asthma, breathing difficulties; use cold externally for insect bites, neuralgia, face pain, pain sensitivity, earache, irritated skin. *Antihistamine, anti-inflammatory, analgesic, vasodilator, bitter, uterine tonic.* Mild reversible side effects in some people include indigestion, diarrhea, nausea, vomiting, nervousness, mouth ulcers, increased bleeding; do not use if allergic to marigolds, ragweed, or chamomile, have a bleeding disorder, are on blood thinners, or are pregnant or nursing; if you stop after long-term use, decrease slowly— withdrawal symptoms of anxiety, headache, muscle stiffness or pain, joint pain, or fatigue may occur.

Flaxseed Oil • *(Linum usitatissimum)*
Also called linseed oil, but linseed products (including paint thinners) are not for ingestion; comes in oil capsules or ground

seed; the ground seed is for use as a bulk laxative, while the oil capsules are used for all other purposes; an essential fatty acid source high in amino acids, fiber, and omega-3 and omega-6 oils; the seed is used for constipation, chronic constipation, bowel inflammatory dis-eases, irritable bowel syndrome, colitis, Crohn's dis-ease, enteritis, colon damage, diverticulitis; balances beneficial bacteria in the intestines, clears the colon of toxins, prevents colon cancer; also reduces stomach acid production, gastritis, soothes ulcers; the oil is an antiestrogen, reducing estrogen by clearing it from the body, important for menopausal symptoms, PMS, cystic breasts, estrogen-sensitive conditions such as fibroid tumors and endometriosis, an aid to preventing and retarding growth of estrogen-sensitive cancers (breast cancer, cervical cancer, ovarian cancer); prevents and treats heart dis-ease and stroke, reduces high blood pressure and high cholesterol, heart pain, angina, and blood clotting; also treats arthritis and rheumatoid arthritis, multiple sclerosis, inflammatory skin dis-eases (psoriasis, eczema, burns, scalds, and irritations); use for obesity; regulates fat in the body, promotes brain development in developing fetuses and in children; reduces inflammation, pain, swelling, pressure

A B C D E F G H I J K L M N O P Q R S T U V W X Y Z

in the eyes, joints, and blood vessels; regulates mucus, water retention, allergic reaction, autonomic nervous system, smooth muscle reflexes, glandular function; lowers blood sugar and may reduce severity of diabetes; regulates immune response. *Antiviral, antibacterial, antifungal, anticancer, antitumor, antioxidant, anti-inflammatory.* Considered a food; no listed side effects, drug interactions, or warnings.

Fo-Ti • *(Polygonum multiflorum)*
Reduces deterioration of aging, primarily for men but with women's uses; must be taken for at least three months for effects to become evident; also called he shou wu or fo-ti shou wu in traditional Chinese medicine; restores vitality, strength, sexual potency, hair growth, and hair color, prevents and treats senility, dizziness, tinnitus, constipation, joint pain, backache; promotes long life and healthy aging; nourishes the liver, kidneys, nervous system, bone marrow, blood circulation; strengthens muscles and bones, tendons and ligaments, brain function, memory, and learning; reduces total and LDL cholesterol, triglycerides; prevents arterial plaque, aids angina, prevents blood clots, increases circulation to the

extremities, reduces fat in the liver, stimulates red blood cell production, prevents and heals infections, increases resistance to dis-ease; immune enhancer; normalizes estrogen levels in women, treats menopausal symptoms and vaginitis, and balances the endocrine system; use externally for skin dis-eases, rashes, wounds, acne, athlete's foot, abrasions, dermatitis, and bruises. *Antioxidant, antifungal, antibacterial, immune booster.* Side effects include cramps, nausea, skin rash, diarrhea, low potassium level; not for use in pregnancy or nursing; can worsen inflammatory bowel dis-eases and liver dis-ease; not for use with diuretics or laxatives.

Garlic • *(Allium sativum)*

Use odor-free in a variety of available products, or eat fresh and uncooked for greatest benefit; prevents, slows, and fights a long list of dis-eases and conditions; immune booster and immune stimulant; protects against free radical damage (antioxidant); can reduce risk of heart dis-ease by 20 to 25 percent and risk of stroke by 30 to 40 percent, reduces high blood pressure, reduces total and LDL cholesterol, increases "good" HDL cholesterol, lowers homocysteine and C-reactive protein (both heart dis-ease markers), prevents blood clots; for diabetes support, lowers blood sugar, increases circulation to the legs and feet, prevents some diabetic complications; increases ability to fight off bacterial and infectious dis-eases; increases resistance to colds, flu, viruses, and infections of all kinds, reduces duration of colds, coughs, flu, croup, bronchitis, earaches, and other respiratory dis-eases (used internally and as a chest rub or in oil as an eardrop); expectorant (thins and expels mucus); formerly used in war to prevent development of gangrene in wounds; may be a preventive and reduces progression of cancer and tumors, including cancers of the colon, stomach, breast, prostate, and throat; reduces chemotherapy side effects and organ damage; expels parasites and intestinal worms; antifungal properties for athlete's foot, nail fungus, *Candida albicans*, thrush; tick repellent; antibacterial against the *H. pylori* bacteria that causes stomach ulcers; cures toothache and gum dis-ease; raises testosterone. *Antioxidant, antiviral, expectorant, anticancer, antiseptic, antimicrobial, antibiotic, antifungal.* Possible side effects include indigestion, bloating, bad breath, body odor, skin irritation; rare side effects of dizziness, headache, fatigue, loss of appetite, muscle aches, skin rash; safe for long-term use; raw garlic used topically can burn the skin; use only food amounts in pregnancy, nursing babies may refuse the breast if mother is taking garlic; use with insulin only on expert advice, and avoid with blood thinners, protease inhibitors, and sulfonylurea drugs.

Gentian Root • *(Gentiana lutea)*

Called yellow gentian, not the same as gentian violet (used for thrush); an ingredient in Angostura Bitters liqueur, and ingredient in many digestive remedies and combinations, including Swedish bitters; easiest to take in capsules (very bitter taste) and usually directed to be taken thirty minutes before eating; fortifier and tonic for all the systems of the body, particularly the digestive and eliminative systems; strengthens the function of liver, gallbladder, stomach acids, spleen, pancreas, kidneys, and circulatory system; for aiding digestion, assimilation of fats; use for indigestion, stomach cramps, too-full heavy feeling after eating, gas, dizziness, diarrhea and constipation, bowel cleansing, including from chronic constipation, toxin and poison antidote, malnourished people including the elderly; increases secretion of digestive juices and liver bile, increases blood supply to the digestive organs (and all the body), aid for digestive weakness; stimulant and tonic for debilitated people; aid for recovery from surgery or with chronic dis-eases, for exhaustion, fatigue, weakness, anemia, lack of appetite, anorexia nervosa; increases energy, strength, endurance, and vitality; expels worms and parasites, and is more effective than quinine for malaria; also for venomous bites (snakes, insects), jaundice, liver inflammation; reduces fever, cools the body, brings on menses, aids reproductive organ weakness in women, eases morning sickness, clears sinus and mucus conditions (usually used with other herbs); use externally to dissolve skin tumors. *Antacid, tonic bitter, anti-inflammatory, liver stimulant, antiseptic.* Not for use by those with excess stomach acid conditions, heartburn, ulcers, gastritis, gastroesophageal reflux dis-ease (GERD); no known drug interactions or side effects.

Ginger • *(Zingiber officinale)*

Root used as tea, tincture, food spice, or chewed fresh, available whole in most supermarkets; use 2 to 4 grams per day; not for children under two years old; best remedy for hiccups, drink 5 to 10 drops of tincture in a tablespoon of water, hiccups stop almost immediately; use for indigestion, upset stomach, heartburn, gas, stomach cramps, diarrhea, belching; primary remedy for nausea and vomiting from all sources: motion and seasickness, morning sickness, chemotherapy, after surgery; aids muscle and joint pain, sprains, arthritis, rheumatism, ulcerative colitis; in heart dis-ease, it lowers cholesterol and prevents blood clots and artery blockage, increases circulation; blood thinner; use for cold and flu symptoms, fever, chills, coughs, sore throat, sinus congestion, sinusitis, headache, migraine, and menstrual cramps; brings on menses. *Analgesic, anti-inflammatory, antibacterial, antiemetic, antispasmodic, stimulant, digestive.* May rarely cause increased heartburn and gas or throat constriction in people allergic to it; not for use by people with bleeding disorders or taking blood thinners (including aspirin), or those with gallstones.

Gingko • *(Gingko biloba)*

Oldest continuing tree species; the herb is helpful for anti-aging, deterioration from aging, and longevity; primarily a blood-vessel dilator and relaxant, makes the blood vessels and red blood cells more flexible to promote circulation; brings more blood nourishment to the heart, brain, and all organs; interferes with PAF (platelet activating factor) that causes asthma attacks and anaphylactic reations; free-radical antioxidant, protects the cells from damage; protects vascular and central nervous systems from deterioration of aging; increases blood flow to the brain and central nervous system to aid stroke recovery, mental clarity, memory, concentration, and cognitive function; treats disorientation, cerebral insufficiency; prevents blood clots, peripheral vascular disease, leg cramps, intermittent claudication, vertigo (dizziness), tinnitus, headaches, depression (especially in elderly and those not responding to depression medications), and all circulatory dis-eases; reduces damage from chemotherapy, radiation therapy, and medications; use for senile dementia, age-related cognitive decline, Alzheimer's dis-ease; improves glaucoma, some deafness, macular degeneration, edema, lung function, coughs, allergies; lowers blood pressure, controls premature aging. *Vasodilator, antioxidant, antiaging.* Takes four to six weeks for benefits to manifest; considered safe for long-term use; possible side effects include indigestion, dizziness, restlessness, diarrhea, headaches, and insomnia; not for use with blood thinners (including aspirin), with blood-clotting disorders or before surgery; not for children, or when pregnant or breastfeeding.

Ginseng, Asian • *(Panax ginseng)*

Korean ginseng, Asian all-healer; *Panax ginseng* is for men and promotes yang energy (Siberian or American ginseng is for women; *see* Ginseng, Siberian); adaptogen (tonic) that promotes endurance and the body's ability to recover from any form of stress; blood cleanser and detoxifier, immune builder; prevents and heals cellular damage; male aphrodisiac and fertility; regulates the central nervous system, improves nerve growth, nerve transmission, mental function, memory, nervous dis-eases, headaches; regulates blood pressure (too high or too low), increases circulation, lowers LDL cholesterol, raises HDL cholesterol, supports efficient heart function and heart recovery from shock; reduces blood sugar, aids diabetes (monitor blood sugar carefully, can induce hypoglycemia); reduces uric acid, kidney stones, gout; use for immune and autoimmune conditions, such as arthritis, lupus, chronic fatigue,

A
B
C
D
E
F
G
H
I
J
K
L
M
N
O
P
Q
R
S
T
U
V
W
X
Y
Z

colds and flu, allergies, bronchitis, asthma, and all infectious dis-eases; physical stamina, stress resistance, adaptation to heat and cold, exhaustion; relaxes muscles and lungs; use for digestion, irritable bowel syndrome, liver function and recovery, hepatitis, cirrhosis; also use for skin conditions (detoxifier), ulcers, eczema, psoriasis, rosacea, rashes, wounds, scars, and for red blood cell production and anemia; anticancer, suppresses cancerous cell growth but is estrogenic and not for women's hormone-dependent cancers or conditions (breast cancer, ovarian cancer, uterine cancer, endometriosis, fibroid tumors) or men's prostate cancer. *Adaptogen, immune enhancer, detoxifier, anticancer, antidepressant, estrogenic.* Should not be used in pregnancy or nursing, for infants or children; overdose can cause restlessness, insomnia, serious hypoglycemic effects (shakiness, confusion), nausea, headaches, diarrhea, internal bleeding, and potentially dangerous too-low or too-high blood pressure; not for use with blood thinners, insulin, high caffeine, and some other medications; start with a very small dose (fewer than 5 drops of tincture) and increase gradually to comfort level; if restlessness or insomnia occurs, reduce dosage or stop; commercially available combined with propolis in a delicious single-dose liquid, and in dry packets that are milder in effect.

Ginseng, Siberian • *(Eleutherococcus senticosus)*

Siberian or American ginseng, yin ginseng for women and women's needs; made popular in 1977 in book *Women and the Crisis in Sex Hormones* by Barbara Seaman and Gideon Seaman, MD, as an alternative to hormone replacement drugs in menopause; fewer and milder side effects with more benefits than *Panax ginseng*; tonic (adaptogen) that strengthens the life force and both body and mind's resistance to stress, depletion, and dis-ease; more useful for sustaining and maintaining good health than for healing dis-ease states; increases longevity, antiaging; reduces or stops menopausal symptoms, especially when used with black cohosh, licorice root, or dong quai; hormone balancer; anticancer, retards cancer cell growth in breast, ovaries, stomach, mouth, and skin; protects the body during radiation and chemotherapy and reduces side effects; immune enhancer that increases production of T-cells, cytotoxic (cancer-killer) cells, and natural killer cells in the immune system; balances high or low blood pressure, lowers high cholesterol, lowers blood sugar (diabetes); central nervous system stimulant; aid for alertness, memory, mental function, emotional disorders; reduces anxiety, depression; aids drug-withdrawal symptoms; increases physical strength and stamina, heals exhaustion and fatigue, including chronic fatigue; adrenal and pituitary nourishment and healing; aids digestion and digestive system dis-eases, liver and kidneys; said to reduce glaucoma and color blindness; also for respiratory system, lungs, colds and flu, bronchitis, headache, insomnia, low back pain, appetite stimulant, arthritis; an all-healer for many conditions. *Adaptogen, tonic, antiaging, anticancer, immune enhancer, hormone balancer.* Side effects include possible insomnia or drowsiness, confusion, vomiting, headache, nosebleed, or irregular heart rhythm; do not use when pregnant or breastfeeding, with children or infants, or with sleep disorders (sleep apnea, narcolepsy); use caution with caffeine and if you have high blood pressure; has probable drug interactions with digoxin and sleep medications; some sources recommend that it not be used continuously for more than three weeks at a time.

Goji Berry • *(Lycium barbarum)*

Good-tasting berry from Tibet and China, called a longevity superfood; eaten as whole berries, dried, or as juice, alone or in cooking; very high in amino acids, plant proteins, vitamins, minerals, and antioxidants; high antioxidant properties protect the cells and all body systems from damage and destruction; repairs the DNA, stimulates HGH (human growth hormone) for weight loss, better sleep, memory enhancement, accelerated healing, youthful appearance, libido; prevents growth of cancer cells; supports the cardiovascular system, reduces high blood pressure, high cholesterol; prevents plaque buildup on arterial walls, increases circulation and blood flow, balances blood sugar (hypoglycemia and diabetes), and reduces sugar cravings; promotes good health, vitality, antiaging, energy, endurance; heals fatigue and debility, aids illness recovery; tonic for the bones and muscles, liver, kidneys, and digestion; stress adaptor, antidepressant; balances women's hormones in menopause; immune stimulant; also for better sleep, dizziness, headaches, infertility (men and women), hyperactivity in children, vision, night vision, macular degeneration; appetite suppressant, aids weight loss. *Antioxidant, adaptogen, anticancer.* No known side effects, warnings, or drug interactions.

Goldenseal • *(Hydrastis canadensis)*

Becoming endangered from overuse and overharvesting; try Oregon grape root or yerba mansa instead and use goldenseal only when no other herb will suffice; herbal sulfa drug, herbal antibiotic; mouth rinse for infected gums and canker sores (especially used with myrrh; try plain myrrh tincture or aloe vera juice instead); boosts the benefits of other herbs; heals sores, wounds, infections, eye infections, mucus conditions; with cayenne pepper in capsules, can prevent or stop a pending cold; use for respiratory infections and congestions of all kinds; traditionally used for serious childhood infectious dis-eases such as scarlet fever, measles, and meningitis; anti-malaria, anticancer; use for uterine infections, cervical dysplasia (douche), herpes blisters (externally), liver dis-eases, gallbladder (stimulates bile production), diabetes (lowers blood sugar); stops profuse bleeding and disinfects cuts and wounds (externally); has grown very popular because its use masks recreational drugs in urine tests. *Antibiotic, antibacterial,*

antiviral, antifungal, tonic, astringent, diuretic, laxative, bitter.
Side effects may include nausea, diarrhea, mood swings, and
photosensitivity; not for continuous or long-term use; can
cause miscarriage, not for use by those with hypoglycemia
(lowers blood sugar), high blood pressure, or heart dis-ease, or
with some blood pressure and blood-thinning medications.

Gotu Kola • *(Centella asiatica)*

Ayurvedic herb also called Indian pennywort; not kola nut—
gotu kola contains no caffeine or caffeine effects; primary
effects are on rejuvenating the mind, brain, and central nervous system; brain tonic, brain food, increases mental function, intelligence, memory, concentration, ability to focus,
ability to meditate, energy replenishment; balances both sides
of the brain, relaxes, reduces fatigue; reduces stress and anxiety, depression, nervous disorders, nervous breakdown, insomnia; use for Alzheimer's dis-ease, senile dementia, children's
ADHD, epilepsy and seizure dis-orders; strengthens the circulatory system, veins, capillaries, arteries; improves blood flow,
reduces high blood pressure (but not high cholesterol or blood
sugar), phlebitis, leg cramps, varicose veins, heavy legs, leg

sores, venous insufficiency, poor circulation; slows retinopathy; encourages new growth of connective tissues and skin, collagen growth, cartilage repair; prevents scarring when used on new wounds, speeds healing time, wound healing, burn healing, including second- and third-degree burns; use for skin and stomach ulcers, skin disorders, psoriasis, hair and nail growth; speeds recovery from surgery; strengthens the adrenals and immune system, clears mucus from the tissues, reduces fevers, destroys tumor cells; diuretic, detoxifier; use for arthritis, sexually transmitted infections, liver dis-eases, hepatitis, and much more. *Tonic, diuretic, detoxifier, immune balancer.* May raise cholesterol and/or blood sugar; side effects: photosensitivity, itching, nausea, indigestion, skin rash; not for use in pregnancy; may interfere or interact negatively with sedative and antipsychotic drugs, diabetes drugs, and cholesterol-reducing drugs.

Grapefruit Seed Extract • *(Citrus paradisi)*

Also called GSE and found in many health food store preparations for washing vegetables and meat, cleaning products, disinfectants, cosmetics, and medicinal preparations; the liquid is very bad tasting but tablets are available; high in vitamin C and potassium, newly introduced in the 1980s whereas most herbals have traditional origins; almost an all-healer with endless uses; antiseptic that destroys bacteria, viruses, fungi, microbes, parasites, protozoa, molds, mildew, and other pathogens; works on strep and staph infections (including some antibiotic-resistant ones), giardia, *E. coli*, herpes, *Salmonella*, *Proteus*, *Klebsiella*, cholera, *Candida albicans*, and more, but doesn't kill beneficial intestinal bacteria as drugs do; corrects intestinal flora levels; used for infections and viruses, vaginitis, and yeast overruns (in a douche), diarrhea and constipation, traveler's dysentery, food poisoning, sore throat (gargle), earaches (in eardrops), indigestion, skin infections (externally), intestinal infections, irritable bowel syndrome; increases resistance and prevents spread of colds, flu, respiratory infections; immune enhancer; increases body utilization of fats and carbohydrates for weight loss; lymphatic drainer, detoxifier; increases the effects of some medications. *Antibacterial, antiviral, antifungal, antibiotic.* No known side effects or warnings, but those allergic to citrus may be allergic to GSE; some drugs are inactivated or made more potent—research yours.

A
B
C
D
E
F
G
H
I
J
K
L
M
N
O
P
Q
R
S
T
U
V
W
X
Y
Z

Grape Seed Extract • *(Vitis vinifera)*

Offers the benefits of red wine without the alcohol; active ingredient is resveratrol, a significant antioxidant that protects the body from free-radical damage; protects the cardiovascular system, keep capillaries from breaking, prevents blood clots, lowers total and LDL cholesterol, increases HDL (good) cholesterol, lowers blood pressure; prevents heart dis-ease, heart attack, and stroke; prevents and helps chronic venous insufficiency, varicose veins, spider veins, phlebitis (blood clots in the legs), leg ulcers; prevents and helps degenerative conditions of the eyes due to blood-vessel deterioration, macular degeneration, light sensitivity, poor night vision, retinopathy, cataracts; prevents and heals hemorrhoids; reduces blood sugar levels for diabetes control, increases insulin uptake, aids acute and chronic pancreatic inflammation; anticancer and antitumor, prevents and stops the growth of cancers of breast, stomach, colon, lungs, prostate, and skin; prevents liver damage from chemotherapy treatment and lessens chemo side effects while increasing effectiveness; may interfere with virus replication in HIV/AIDS; also for allergies and allergic reactions, asthma, obesity (blocks absorption of fat); prevents internal and external scarring, reduces tooth decay, heals the skin, promotes healing and regeneration of connective tissue, prevents cellular damage; mood stabilizer. *Antioxidant, antitumor, anticancer, antiviral.* Side effects may include stomach cramps, sore throat, cough, headache, diarrhea, nausea; avoid in pregnancy, breastfeeding, and for children; avoid with blood-thinning drugs, including aspirin.

Green Tea • *(Camellia sinensis)*

Widely known in Asia for thousands of years but relatively new to the West; green tea is a major antioxidant and anti-inflammatory in a tasty, inexpensive beverage; requires four or more cups per day to have effect; teas are more effective than capsules, contains caffeine (about 40 mg per cup; caffeinated coffee contains 85 mg per cup) but decaffeinated green teas and green tea capsules are available; primary cancer fighter for breast, prostate, lung, stomach, skin, and esophagus; reduces rate of cancer growth, kills cancer cells, shrinks tumors, helps protect organs from cancer, helps prevent recurrence after cancer treatment, heals skin damaged by radiation therapy; aids digestion, abdominal bloating;

raises metabolism for weight loss (probably too little to be significant), normalizes beneficial bacteria in intestines; reduces food poisoning, bad breath, gum dis-ease, tooth decay, and dental plaque by killing the bacteria that cause them; prevents heart dis-ease and stroke by reducing arterial inflammation and blood clot formation, lowers total cholesterol levels, and improves the ratio between HDL (good) and LDL (bad) cholesterol; immune booster; reduces inflammation in all organs; use for rheumatoid arthritis, infections, wound healing, blotchy skin, and skin cancer (use externally in a skin cream); controls bleeding, regulates body temperature, aids diabetes (by reducing blood sugar), promotes urinary tract and brain function, relieves thirst, slows aging; slows the progression of neurological dis-eases, including Parkinson's dis-ease, multiple sclerosis, Alzheimer's disease, and AIDS. *Antioxidant, antibacterial, antiviral, antiaging, anticancer, anti-inflammatory.* Mild possible caffeine side effects (avoid by using decaffeinated forms): indigestion, appetite loss, constipation or diarrhea, nervousness, irritability, insomnia, headache, palpitations; caution if pregnant or with hyperthyroid dis-ease, high blood pressure, kidney dis-ease, blood clotting disorder, or if using blood thinners, pseudoephedrine, or other drugs.

Grindelia • *(Grindelia robusta)*

Atropine-like effects to first increase heart rate then lower it, first increase blood pressure then lower it; specific remedy for asthmatic breathing, breathlessness from heart dis-ease, irregular heart action with accompanying cough; in spasmodic coughs, it stops the coughing reflex then breaks up and expels mucus; soothes bronchial irritation, eases dry spasmodic coughs, chronic cough after pneumonia, whooping cough, asthma, bronchitis, hay fever; must be given in repeated small doses to have effect but can effect a permanent cure; external use for inflamed and irritated skin; antidotes poison ivy and poison oak, burns, insect bites, rashes, blisters, skin infections, skin ulcers, wounds that don't heal; also use for cystitis, urinary tract irritation and infection. *Antispasmodic, expectorant, sedative.* Must be used in small doses; overdose can result in dangerous respiratory paralysis; may irritate stomach and kidneys, and cause frequent urination; no known drug interactions or warnings except not to overdose; considered safe with normal use.

Guarana • *(Paullina cupona)*

Guarana is the popular caffeine beverage drink of Brazil, used in commercial cola-type drinks, chewed, or the powder diluted in water; contains 160 mg of caffeine per teaspoon, which is two or three times the amount of caffeine in coffee; used as coffee is used in North America, as a stimulant and to overcome fatigue; touted for weight loss and included in several weight-loss combination formulas, in athletic preparations to increase endurance and stamina, and as a remedy for migraines and headaches (some migraines will respond to American caffeinated colas, too); also a tonic, diuretic, pain reliever, fever reducer, antiseptic, detoxifier, sexual enhancer, antidepressant, antiasthmatic; central nervous system stimulant, enhances alertness, energy, long-term memory, masks fatigue and exhaustion, debility, jet lag, and hangover; also for amnesia, nerve pain, neuralgia, rheumatism, heat stroke; increases blood sugar levels for hypoglycemia from hard exercise (not for diabetic use); blood thinner, prevents and clears blood clots, high cholesterol, high blood pressure; dilates the blood vessels, stimulates and strengthens the heart; aids digestion, indigestion, gas, constipation but also used for diarrhea, chronic diarrhea, and dysentery; brings on menses, reduces water retention, PMS, cramps; mood raiser; douche for vaginal infections; used in cosmetics for oily hair and skin, cellulite, hair loss, skin disorders; antibacterial, kills *E. coli* and *Salmonella*. *Antioxidant, stimulant, vasodilator, diuretic, antibacterial, astringent, adaptogen.* Nontoxic even long term and at high doses; do not use if caffeine intolerant, if pregnant or nursing, or with high blood pressure, heart dis-ease, epilepsy, diabetes, stomach ulcers, chronic headache, or where increased heat is not wanted; avoid if taking blood thinners.

Gymnema • *(Gymnema sylvestre)*

Ayurvedic plant also called gurmar, or "sugar destroyer," primary use is for control of blood sugar levels in diabetes; takes three to four weeks for benefits to start, and may take six months to two years for full benefit; controls blood sugar levels for type 1 and type 2 diabetics without hypoglycemic effects (without reducing too far); improves body's response to insulin; raises insulin levels in the blood by regenerating pancreatic beta (insulin-producing) cells; decreases the amount of sugar absorbed from food by up to 50 percent;

stops sugar cravings and the ability to taste sweets for three hours after use; may decrease need for insulin by 45 to 75 percent; reduces insulin resistance, cholesterol and triglycerides; reduces the absorption of dietary fat from the intestines into the bloodstream, protects the liver, and promotes weight loss. *Antidiabetic*. Can be used long term; has no side effects but hypoglycemic reactions are possible; insulin and blood sugar levels must be monitored carefully, diabetic medications may have to be reduced.

Hawthorn • *(Crataegeus oxycantha, Crataegeus species)*
Very safe natural heart strengthener that can be used long term and taken with most heart and blood pressure medications; strengthens heart and cardiovascular function, aids weak and damaged hearts, reduces incidence of strokes and heart attacks; heart nutrient, heart tonic; reduces high blood pressure, increases flow of blood and oxygen to and from the heart, relaxes and dilates arteries, protects arteries from developing plaque (atherosclerosis), removes LDL cholesterol from bloodstream, reduces cholesterol production in the liver, increases strength and endurance; use for cardiac insufficiency, palpitations from

heart dis-ease or menopause, arrhythmia, angina, shortness of breath, and hypertension in diabetics; promotes and supports healthy circulation, heart and blood vessels; a vasodilator, beta blocker, anti-inflammatory, and antioxidant; also used for indigestion, kidney stones, sore throat, depression, nervousness, insomnia, arthritis, joint pain and stiffness. *Vasodilator, heart tonic, diuretic, astringent, anti-inflammatory, antioxidant, antispasmodic.* Rare side effects include headache, rash, nausea, dizziness, sweating, agitation, or palpitations; not for use in pregnancy or for children under twelve; may interfere with digoxin or other heart medicines.

Hibiscus Flower • *(Hibiscus rosa-sinensis)*

Beautiful flowers, easy to grow in the South; good-tasting beverage tea (add mint for a different taste), high in vitamin C, no caffeine; lowers high blood pressure, lowers LDL cholesterol, inhibits the binding of cholesterol to artery walls, increases blood circulation, helps reduce heart dis-ease and strokes; promising as a treatment for type 1 juvenile diabetes; reduces gallbladder pressure; laxative; stops conversion of carbohydrates to fats, lessens appetite, and promotes weight loss; stops bleeding, reduces heavy menstrual bleeding and menstrual cramps, eases spasms and cramps throughout the body; soothes the mucous membranes of the respiratory tract, antibacterial for respiratory infections, coughs, whooping cough; reduces fever; soothes the digestive system, aids poor digestion, indigestion; diuretic, pain reliever; use for cystitis; traditional for sexually transmitted infections; external wash for the skin. *Astringent, analgesic, antispasmodic, diuretic, antibacterial.* The dried herb is best when kept no longer than six months; avoid with gallstones; no other known side effects, warnings, or drug interactions.

Holy Basil • *(Ocimum sanctum)*

Hindu sacred herb also called tulsi; stress adaptor, free-radical scavenger; balances the mind, nerves, and emotions; protects from pollutants and toxins, including dental mercury; immune stimulant, reduces all inflammations; nourishes the adrenals, heart, and central nervous system; expectorant for respiratory mucus conditions, chest congestion, wet coughs; use for colds, flu, sore throat, viral and bacterial infections, asthma, allergies, tuberculosis, fever, earache, night blindness; used in many cough syrups and flu preparations; aids digestion by increasing digestive enzymes, increases appetite; use for indigestion, gas, diarrhea, dysentery, children's upset stomachs, vomiting, urinary infections, hepatitis, headaches; brings out pending chicken pox or measles; strengthens the heart, lowers blood sugar, and improves beta cell function for diabetics; laxative, poison antidote, blood cleanser, menstrual regulator, arthritis and cancer preventive, pain reliever; for stress-related skin conditions; used externally with castor oil for head lice. *Adaptogen, antibacterial, antiparasitic, antioxidant, anti-inflammatory, expectorant, antiviral.* Never drink milk right after taking holy basil; do not ingest the essential oil; not for use in pregnancy, nursing, or when trying to conceive; seek expert advice with kidney or liver dis-ease; no known side effects or drug interactions.

Hoodia Gordonii • *(Asclipiadaceae gordonii)*

African succulent plant used by bushmen of the Kalahari desert; endangered plant that requires both a USDA permit and a CITES certificate to export; there are more than 300 hoodia products being advertised and it's estimated that 80 percent are fraudulent (that is, they do not contain hoodia gordonii;

only the gordonii form of hoodia contains the active P57 ingredient; attempts to synthesize P57 by big pharmaceutical companies have so far proved toxic or failed; appetite suppressant that makes the brain think it's full even when it's not; used by indigenous people to suppress hunger and thirst when hunting in the desert; reduces blood sugar (hypoglycemic) but also suppresses low blood sugar warning symptoms; also used for indigestion, minor infections, high blood pressure, depression; used to increase energy and as an aphrodisiac; may be a hope for seriously obese people but not without caution; may take several weeks to show benefit. *Hypoglycemic, appetite suppressant.* No evident side effects, but synthesized versions are liver toxic and may be fatal; not for use by diabetics, with hypoglycemia, kidney dis-ease, or if pregnant or nursing; drug interactions still unknown; buyers beware, as many preparations do not contain the herb.

Hops • *(Humulus lupulus, Lupuli strobulus)*
Ingredient and flavoring in beer making; used medicinally since early Egypt, written documentation of medicinal use in Germany in 822 CE; primarily used as a sedative and

calmative, also a stomach tonic, blood cleanser, liver cleanser, and stimulant; sedates the central nervous system to help relieve insomnia, restlessness, anxiety, nervousness, stress, mood upsets, delirium tremens, convulsions, neuralgia, nerve pain; also used as a general pain reliever; as a stomach tonic and bitter, stimulates production of gastric juices, aids digestive assimilation, indigestion, improves appetite, heartburn; cleanses and stimulates the liver; use for liver dis-eases and jaundice; reduces bowel inflammation, dysentery, Crohn's dis-ease, irritable bowel syndrome; expels intestinal worms and parasites; bladder cleanser, diuretic; use for cystitis, irritable bladder, urinary gravel, kidney stones, kidney infections and dis-eases; estrogenic effects for menopausal symptoms, hot flashes, osteoporosis, breast enhancer; used in heart disease to lower cholesterol and triglycerides, and as a calmative; blood cleanser; may be antiherpes, anti–Epstein Barr (chronic fatigue), antirhinovirus (respiratory virus conditions, colds), anti-HIV; used dry in a pillow for toothache, earache, nervousness, insomnia (especially with valerian); as a poultice combined with chamomile or poppy for swelling, inflammation, neuralgia, rheumatism pain, muscle spasms, skin

A
B
C
D
E
F
G
H
I
J
K
L
M
N
O
P
Q
R
S
T
U
V
W
X
Y
Z

ulcers, bruises, and boils. *Antispasmodic, antiviral, diuretic, digestive bitter, antibacterial, anti-inflammatory, sedative, astringent, antiseptic.* Possible side effects found mostly in hops harvesters of contact allergy, drowsiness, increased or decreased blood sugar levels; contains phytoestrogens that may interact unfavorably with hormone-sensitive cancers and conditions; suspected drug interactions (have not been studied) with diabetic drugs (raised or lowered blood sugar), hormones (may increase effects of hormone replacement therapy, estrogens), sedative and antipsychotic drugs (may increase effects); generally considered safe.

Horehound • *(Marrubium vulgare)*

Also called white horehound; used commercially in many cough syrups and expectorants; clears the lungs of phlegm (thins mucus); use for coughs, lung infections, wheezing, asthma, colds, sore throat, bronchitis, whooping cough, pneumonia, shortness of breath, croup, tuberculosis, chronic obstructive pulmonary dis-ease (COPD); reduces fever; also a pain reliever, stomach tonic, liver and gallbladder stimulant, bile stimulant, laxative in larger doses, antitumor, diuretic;

use for jaundice, liver dis-eases, indigestion, gas, heartburn, bloating, overfullness, loss of appetite, intestinal dis-eases; expels worms; lowers blood pressure, reduces heart arrhythmia in normal doses, reduces blood sugar; use for diabetes, water retention; brings on menses, stimulates menstrual flow, abortifacient in early pregnancy when used as hot tea; used externally for wounds, herpes sores, shingles, eczema. *Antispasmodic, antioxidant, diuretic, expectorant, stimulant, tonic, antibacterial, antitumor.* Side effects include disturbed heart rhythm, low blood pressure, low blood sugar, vomiting, diarrhea, contact dermatitis; also a strong bile stimulant; increases stomach acid; not for use with low blood pressure, hypoglycemia, pregnancy, stomach ulcers, gastroesophageal reflux dis-ease (GERD); caution with heart dis-ease, diabetes, gastrointestinal dis-eases; may interact with tuberculosis drugs, blood sugar regulators, and more—research your medications carefully.

Horse Chestnut • *(Aesculus hippocastanum)*
Known to many children as buckeye tree; only the processed extracts and remedies are safe for use—the fresh herb is liver

112

toxic; primary use is for chronic venous insufficiency that includes varicose veins, spider veins, swollen legs and ankles, leg cramps, especially at night, phlebitis (blood clots), itching skin, skin ulcers, and heavy, tired, dragging legs; tones the vein walls, increases circulation to the legs, tightens the veins and other blood vessels, increases blood flow to the legs, prevents blood vessel leakage, and prevents blood clots; also for hemorrhoids, neuralgia, tinnitus, bruising, fractures, swelling, tendonitis, joint and muscle swelling, sprains, soft tissue swelling after surgery; supports vein healing and circulation in brain traumas, strokes, and some heart dis-eases; relieves congested uterus, cervix, and portal veins, lowers blood sugar; diuretic for water retention and edema in PMS, rheumatism, cystitis, urinary gravel, kidney infection and kidney stones, urinary incontinence; reduces intermittent fevers. *Astringent, anti-inflammatory, diuretic, protects the vascular system.* Side effects with processed remedies may include allergy, itching, nausea, indigestion, headache, muscle spasms, dizziness, skin rash, or diarrhea; do not use unprocessed herb; avoid in pregnancy and breastfeeding, with children, or when taking blood thinners, including aspirin.

Horseradish • *(Armoracia rusticana)*

The "bitter herb" of Passover Seders, known today as a hot food condiment; use medicinally by eating a very small amount with food or in a cup of water; increases blood flow in the sinuses and nasal passages, clears upper respiratory congestion, mild antibiotic for upper respiratory infections, coughs, flu, whooping cough; can be used in cough syrups and as a chest poultice; poultices are also used for sore muscles and joints, rheumatism, gout, sciatica, swollen liver or spleen, neuralgia, or frostbite to dilate blood vessels, making skin red and tissues warm; horseradish concentrates in the urine and is used in drugs for bladder infections (cystitis), prevents toxins from remaining in the bladder; diuretic action flushes bladder of infection and may also flush out cancer cells, relieve swelling, bloating, and edema; stimulates digestive system, increases appetite, aids indigestion; stimulates the nervous system, expels intestinal worms, decreases thyroid production. *Bitter, stimulant, diuretic, antiseptic, antigas, rubefacient, laxative.* Overdose side effects include bloody diarrhea or vomit, heavy perspiration, indigestion, or skin blisters and burns with poultices; not for use in pregnancy, breastfeeding, or with children under four years old; can irritate the gastrointestinal tract, may worsen ulcers, kidney disease, or low thyroid; should not be used with blood thinners or thyroid drugs.

Horsetail Grass • *(Equisetum arvense)*

High in silica, rich in calcium and minerals, increases white blood cells, prevents plaque in the arteries, stops slow-bleeding conditions; mainly used as a nutrient, strengthener, and repair-replacement for skin, hair, finger- and toenails, bones, tendons, ligaments, eyes, and cell walls; builds collagen, connective tissue strengthener; remedy for calcium deficiency, increases bone density; used for healing broken bones, bone injuries, torn internal and connective tissue, tendonitis, torn muscle tissue, osteoporosis, sports injuries, back injuries, joint erosion in arthritis, brittle nails, rheumatism, sores, lifeless hair; diuretic to reduce water retention, edema (swelling), bladder and urinary infections, urinary incontinence, bedwetting, swollen legs, diabetes, increases urinary output; stops passive (slow) bleeding internally and externally for blood in the urine (kidney and bladder infections), nosebleeds, ulcers, wounds, tuberculosis, emphysema; use for bleeding of nose, stomach, intestines, lungs, and bronchi; reduces heat, swelling, bleeding, inflammation, and fluid throughout the body for prostate inflammation, intestinal inflammatory disorders, hemorrhoids, dysentery, flu, frostbite, fluid in the lungs, conjunctivitis, corneal abrasions of the eyes, wounds, fevers; may be the best possible remedy for acne, eczema, and psoriasis, used internally and externally; enhances the immune system, protects the liver, balances the thyroid, may be antitumor, clears the body of lead toxicity. *Diuretic, astringent, antibiotic, blood clotting, antibacterial, wound healer.* Safe at normal dose, can cause skin rash; overuse can cause serious thiamine (B_1) deficiency and nicotine overdose symptoms; avoid if B_1 deficient, alcoholic, poor nutrition; not for children, for pregnant or nursing women, or if using diuretic drugs.

Hyssop • *(Hyssopus officinalis)*

Good herb for all excess mucus and fluid conditions, expectorant; use for upper respiratory infections, cold symptoms, sinusitis, cough, chronic cough, pulmonary dis-eases, bronchitis, asthma, laryngitis, pharyngitis, tonsillitis; soothes upper respiratory tract and brings up phlegm; aids food digestion, stomach cramps, colic, gas; in diabetes, prevents spikes in blood sugar levels after eating; use internally and externally (in baths) for rheumatism and aching muscles; as a bath or wash for discolored bruises, cuts, burns, acne, itching skin conditions; and internally and as a gargle for sore throats; may inhibit growth of the HIV virus; also mild sedative; use for headaches, menstrual cramps, and for blood cleansing; traditionally used for purification of sacred sites and as a strewing herb for deodorizing and purifying. *Expectorant, antispasmodic, sedative, antiviral, antigas, antibiotic, diuretic, stimulant, anti-inflammatory.* Not for use in pregnancy or breastfeeding; the essential oil may cause seizures and is not for internal use; no known side effects, warnings, or drug interactions with the herb.

Iceland Moss • *(Cetraria islandica)*

Technically a lichen used for both food and medicine, unique in combining lubrication and soothing with digestive bitter properties; central use is for respiratory infections and breathing disorders, infections with inflammation and dryness, swollen lymph glands, expectorant to thin and expel mucus, for colds, dry hacking coughs, bronchitis, mouth and throat infections, hoarseness, sinusitis; use internally and as a chest poultice, may be used after nasal surgery or hospital intubations to soothe and heal; cellular regenerator, detoxifier, cleanser, and tonic; useful in debilitated people, inhibits the TB bacillus, inhibits viral replication in HIV/AIDS; also for digestive tract infections, food poisoning (inhibits *Salmonella*), gastroenteritis, gastritis, nausea and vomiting, heartburn, anemia, appetite loss; use for kidney and bladder infections, cystitis, trichomonal vaginal infection (douche); stimulates breast milk, expels intestinal worms; external use for infected wounds, skin ulcers, skin growths, impetigo, boils, and abscesses; good used with black horehound for nausea and vomiting. *Expectorant, antiviral, antioxidant, antibiotic, lubricant, digestive bitter.* Possible side effects of diarrhea, gastric irritation, or liver symptoms; must be prepared properly to be safe; for short-term use, do not overdose; not for those with gastric ulcers; no information available on pregnancy or breastfeeding use; no known drug interactions.

Isatis Leaf • *(Isatis tinctoria)*

Also called blue woad, indigowoad, or, in traditional Chinese medicine, ban lan gen; remedy for toxic heat and infectious viral and bacterial dis-eases; used for flu, sore throat, fever, measles, mumps, scarlet fever, syphilis, strep throat, head-aches, laryngitis, carbuncles, encephalitis, coughing blood, eruption dis-eases, high fevers and convulsions in children, and epidemic fever dis-eases; preventive for hepatitis A, certain cancers, meningitis, inflammations; cools the body, detoxi-fies, enhances immune function; used externally for sores and ulcers, heat rash, skin inflammations, as a plaster or poultice for enlarged spleen, and as a salve for bleeding. *Antibacterial, antiviral, anti-inflammatory, astringent, anticancer.* Side effects of allergy and dizziness, may be liver toxic if badly overdosed long term; no drug interactions listed.

Ivy Leaf • *(Hedera helix)*

This is **not** poison ivy, and ivy leaf essential oil is **not** for inter-nal use; improves air flow through the bronchial passages and lungs, keeps airways free of constriction, opens swollen bronchial airways; used for acute or chronic inflammatory bronchial conditions, bronchitis, bronchial spasms, bronchial asthma, whooping cough, chronic obstructive pulmonary disease (COPD), colds, flu, coughs, shortness of breath, spitting of blood; reduces inflammation and congestion; antibacterial, astringent, expectorant; thins mucus, reduces fever, relieves pain; used for dysentery, jaundice, gout, rheumatism; external use in cosmetic preparations for stretch marks, cellulite, sunburn, freckles, warts, and for skin eruptions, itching, eczema, lice, burns, impetigo, neuralgia, swollen joints, toothache, frostbite; helps other ingredients be absorbed through the skin, detoxifies the skin; also used in weight-loss formulas. *Expectorant, astringent, antispasmodic, antibacterial, antifungal.* Rare possible overdose effects include irritability, nausea, vomiting, skin allergy, destruction of red blood cells; not for use in pregnancy, may cause uterine contractions; no known drug interactions.

Jewelweed • *(Impatiens capensis)*

Wherever there is poison ivy, jewelweed grows nearby in wet shady ground; crush a fresh leaf and spread the plant juice on poison ivy or poison oak as an antidote; also available in tinctures and as the major ingredient in a number of anti-poison ivy soaps and salves, including the well-known Sting Stop salve; works by removing the poison ivy irritant chemical urushiol from the skin; used as a wash or in the shower can prevent poison ivy rash from developing, also prevents erupted rash from spreading and antidotes and heals it rapidly; used externally on a variety of skin irritants, including poison oak, stinging nettle, okra plant, bee stings, wasp bites, mosquito bites, all irritating plants, and for acne, ringworm, athlete's foot, heat rash, razor burn, herpes sores, blisters, hemorrhoids, and all dermatitis; protects from ultraviolet sun rays; used traditionally in childbirth as a vaginal wash, and as a skin wash for measles. *Skin healer, poison ivy antidote.* Not recommended for internal use; no side effects, drug interactions, or warnings with topical use.

Juniper Berry • *(Juniperus communis)*

Do not use juniper oil internally or juniper tar at all; juniper berry is used for indigestion from low stomach acid and as a diuretic to flush the kidneys; stimulates production of stomach acid for indigestion, gas, poor appetite, gastrointestinal bacteria and parasites; inactivates the *H. pylori* bacteria that causes stomach ulcers, slows growth of food-poisoning organisms, can slow growth of cancer cells in the stomach and gastrointestinal tract; mild diuretic for water retention, bloating, PMS, urinary tract infections, kidney infections, urinary and kidney stones, gout, rheumatism; for diabetes, lowers blood sugar, increases insulin production in the body for better sugar utilization; abortifacient; external uses include skin rashes, burns, sunburn, minor wounds, scrapes, skin fungus and parasites, skin inflammation, neuralgia; the oil is used for sore muscles and joints as liniment only; in a steam kettle for bronchial congestion and lung inflammation; in the bath for arthritis; in hair rinse for hair loss; not for use in the mouth. *Diuretic, anti-inflammatory, antiseptic, antirheumatic, digestive, antibacterial.* Side effects include kidney irritation, skin rash or skin irritation, breathing difficulty, stomach irritation, and discolored urine; not for use when trying to get pregnant, in pregnancy or breast feeding; not for those with hypoglycemia; diabetics need to monitor blood sugar levels carefully; not for those with excess acid stomach disorders such as gastroesophageal reflux dis-ease (GERD); may interact with diuretic drugs and others—research your medication before using; do not use for longer than four weeks at a time; do not overdose.

Kava Kava • *(Piper methysticum)*

Known in Hawaii and the South Pacific for three thousand years as a safe, nonaddictive social beverage and intoxicant; recent FDA claims of liver toxicity seem unfounded with only kava kava use; 2 kava kava capsules with 2 aspirin taken at the beginning of a migraine will often stop it; tincture is bad tasting, use capsules; elevates mood, relaxes, sedates, relieves pain, offers a sense of wellness and peace, improves mental function, improves concentration, lessens the side effects of some antipsychotic drugs; use for insomnia, anxiety, nervousness, stress; useful for those who are depressed because of cancer or other serious illnesses; helpful for menopausal anxiety and PMS; muscle relaxant; reduces seizures, muscle spasms, back pain, headaches, and migraines; traditionally used for gonorrhea, chronic cystitis (diuretic), gout, rheumatism, dropsy, vaginal infection, colds, bronchitis, and bedwetting; use externally for fungal infections, stings, skin inflammation, local anesthetic. *Aphrodisiac, anesthetic, antiseptic, diuretic, antifungal, antidepressant*. Side effects may include drowsiness, dizziness, restlessness, tremors, or upset stomach; caution says the herb is not for overuse, long-term use, for children, or for those with alcoholism or impaired liver function; may interfere with some medical drugs, especially seizures drugs, antipsychotics, L-dopa for Parkinson's dis-ease, and alcohol.

Kelp • *(Ascophyllum nodosom)*

Canadian or Norwegian kelp is a seaweed or sea vegetable nutritionally high in minerals and iodine, vitamins, omega-3 essential fatty acids, trace elements, growth hormones, enzymes, and proteins; enhances glandular activity, raises metabolism by increasing thyroid hormone production, also detoxifies, nourishes, and causes cellular regeneration; beneficial to brain tissues, sensory nerves, spinal cord, membranes surrounding the brain; use for low thyroid function, goiter, endocrine balance; circulatory system strengthening, artery health, heart dis-ease prevention; helps lower risk of stoke, reduces high blood pressure, reduces high cholesterol; use for respiratory dis-eases, asthma, gastrointestinal disorders, chronic constipation, infectious dis-eases, menopausal support; also for weight loss, obesity, arthritis, rheumatism, bones, nails, skin disorders, teeth; makes hair healthy, prevents and restores hair loss; increases endurance, prevents ulcers, may be anticancer; removes radiation from the body (including from cancer therapy), removes heavy metal toxicity from the body, detoxifies, and a general tonic. *Antibiotic, antiseptic, diuretic, hormone balancer, detoxifier, tonic.* Side effects include interference with thyroid function, irregular heartbeat, pounding heart, nervousness, insomnia, difficulty breathing, excessive fatigue, bleeding, cramps, acne, itching, rash; metallic taste in the mouth and sores at the mouth corners may indicate overuse; not for use in pregnancy or breastfeeding without expert advice; interacts with several kinds of drugs—research yours.

Khella • *(Ammi visnaga)*

Stops spasms in smooth muscle, and dilates blood vessels, urinary tract, and bronchial passages; strengthens a weak heart, increases blood flow to the heart, and relaxes heart arteries without reducing blood pressure, prevents blood clots, prevents blood vessel constriction; helps angina, coronary insufficiency, spastic heart, cardiac asthma; increases ratio of HDL to LDL cholesterol, reduces arterial plaque, lessens risk of heart attack and stroke, aids recovery after heart attack or stroke; relaxes the urinary passages to pass kidney stones, reduces pain of passage, heals irritated tissues after passage of stones, and relieves gallbladder colic and spasm; dilates the bronchial airways for spastic coughs, bronchitis, emphysema, asthma; prevents and reduces frequency of asthma attacks; also relieves stomach cramps, PMS, and menstrual cramps; external use for skin wounds, psoriasis, vitiligo, and inflammatory skin conditions. *Antispasmodic, vasodilator.* Requires long-term use for benefit; overdose effects include photosensitivity, nausea, headache, insomnia, liver congestion; avoid in pregnancy, while breastfeeding, or when taking blood thinners; may interfere with effectiveness of heart medications; expert advice recommended in cases of high blood pressure or heart dis-ease.

Kudzu Root • *(Pueraria lobata, Pueraria montana)*
Imported plant that has become an invasive and expensive pest along America's Southeastern highways; used in traditional

Chinese medicine since 200 BCE; also called arrowroot; an herbal Antabuse for alcohol addiction, take 2 capsules with an alcoholic beverage and illness (nausea and hangover) comes while still drinking; used for alcohol withdrawal support, prevents alcohol addiction, stops alcohol cravings, heals hangover; also used for headaches, migraines, cluster migraines, tinnitus, and vertigo; relieves pain; use for colds, flu, sinusitis, fever with chills, nausea; breaks out pending measles or chicken pox infections, treats convulsions; treats inflammatory skin conditions and dermatitis; prevents heart dis-ease by increasing blood supply to the heart; circulatory stimulant, vasodilator; protects the capillaries, stabilizes heart rhythm, aids angina, reduces blood pressure; prevents cancer and leukemia. *Antispasmodic, anti-inflammatory, antimicrobial, anticancer, diuretic, antioxidant, vascular protector.* Possible side effects include mild temporary anemia and elevated liver enzymes; seek expert advice with medications or preexisting conditions; not for use in pregnancy or breastfeeding, with diabetes or hypoglycemia.

Lady's Mantle • *(Alchemilla vulgaris)*

Use internally and externally to stop bleeding and heal wounds; use for internal and external wounds, inflammation, sores, bleeding, infections, mouth sores (apthous ulcers); drying and astringent, soothing, relieves pain; also for acne, conjunctivitis (dilute tea as eyewash), laryngitis and sore throat (gargle), diarrhea, vomiting, spasms, convulsions; in a sleep pillow to promote sleep, in a steam bath for complexion toning; notable use for menopause and menstruation, excessive menstrual bleeding; regulates cycles, reduces cramps and symptoms of PMS, brings on menses, contracts the uterus, heals vaginitis, reduces fibroid tumors, heals soreness after childbirth; use as a diuretic for cystitis, water retention, edema, weight gain from water retention; regulates circulation, protects the circulatory system, increases vein elasticity, prevents and clears phlebitis (blood clots), varicose veins, spider veins, high cholesterol, and high blood pressure. *Astringent, anti-inflammatory, antibacterial, diuretic, wound healer, uterine tonic.* Not for use in pregnancy or with stomach ulcers; seek expert advice with heart dis-ease, high blood pressure, liver dis-ease; no known side effects or drug interactions.

Lavender • *(Lavendula angustifolia)*

Most often used as an external-only essential oil, but the flowers and leaves may be taken internally as an herbal tea. Dried flowers stuffed in herb pillows are used for insomnia, relaxation, stress, calming, headaches, depression, and pain relief; the tea is a relaxing bedtime drink for comfortable sleep; quiets the body and the mind, antidepressant, antistress, nerve tonic, gives a feeling of overall peace and well-being; may be useful for agitated behavior, dementia, and Alzheimer's disease; also for colic, gas, heartburn, headaches and migraines, nervous stomach, hangover, fever, exhaustion, faintness, menstrual cramps, pain; appetite stimulant, mild diuretic; use as a gargle for sore throat, hoarseness, and laryngitis; use lavender essential oil externally in baths, sprinkled on pillows, or heated in water in an aromatherapy lamp for insomnia, headaches, relaxation, circulatory stimulation, pain, faintness, dizziness, fatigue and exhaustion, colic, palpitations, spasms, colds, fever, menopausal symptoms, asthma, bronchitis; use topically for skin dis-eases, alopecia (hair loss disease), eczema, acne, sores, burns, diaper rash, muscle spasms, sprains, arthritis, carpal tunnel syndrome, varicose veins, and much more. *Antidepressant, antibacterial, antispasmodic, anti-inflammatory, antifungal, nerve tonic, antigas.* Though rare, oil (not for internal use) or herb can be an allergen; side effects include hormonal imbalance, drowsiness, confusion, nausea, vomiting, headache, chills, changes in appetite, constipation; not for use in pregnancy or breastfeeding; may increase the effects of sedative and antianxiety medications.

Lemon Balm • *(Melissa officinalis)*

Also called balm, a cooking and culinary herb of the mint family; use fresh or in tea, capsules, or tinctures, but the essential oil is not for internal use; primarily used as an antidepressant and calmative; use for stress, insomnia, nervousness, nerve disorders, emotional upset, tension, anxiety, agitation, hypochondria; promotes calm alertness, sense of well-being; reduces dizziness, fainting, seizures, headaches and migraines, nervous indigestion, gas; muscle relaxant; may be useful for Alzheimer's dis-ease, ADHD, hyperthyroid conditions, and is possibly anti-HIV; induces sweating to break fevers, clears mucus from the lungs, decongestant for colds, flu, sore throats, minor viruses; antihistamine, reduces congestion and allergic reactions; used for PMS, menstrual cramps, brings on menses; also used as a heart and circulatory tonic; lowers blood pressure, soothes intestinal dis-eases; topical cleanser for wounds and sores, used traditionally for scorpion, snake, and animal bites; it is being investigated for herpes sores. *Antibacterial, antiviral, antidepressant, antispasmodic, antioxidant, calmative, breaks fever.* No reported side effects, toxicities, or warnings; do not use the oil internally; may interfere with sedatives and thyroid drugs.

Licorice Root • *(Glycyorhiza glabra)*

Familiar food and candy flavoring, though most "licorice" is anise today, contains more sweetness than sugar; use DGL (deglycyrrhizinated) form to prevent side effects; best herbal ulcer and bleeding ulcer remedy, an herbal hydrocortisone; promotes hormone and glandular balance, increases efficiency of liver and kidneys, helps hot flashes and menopausal symptoms; antacid effective for gastric reflux, immune stimulant, deactivates viruses, and lowers cholesterol; external use for herpes, heals lesions faster and prevents recurrence; useful externally for all skin conditions, soothing and healing; use for adrenal exhaustion, Addison's dis-ease, polycystic ovary syndrome, asthma, viral infections, hepatitis and liver dis-eases, arthritis, all inflammations, chronic fatigue, fever, sore throats, respiratory dis-eases, bladder infections, indigestion, mouth sores, weight loss, anemia, diabetes, allergic reactions and allergies. *Antibacterial, antioxidant, expectorant, anti-inflammatory, laxative, antispasmodic, anticancer, adrenal tonic.* Side effects (high blood pressure, salt and water retention, low potassium, heart dis-ease) are mostly avoided by using DGL licorice; avoid use with diuretic drugs and steroids; avoid if pregnant, or with high blood pressure or renal failure; use con-tinuously no longer than four to six weeks.

Linden Flower • *(Tillia cordata)*

Also called lime blossom or tillia; combines well with cham-omile for all uses, hawthorn for heart support; commercial extracts are available that combine the linden flower with mis-tletoe for high blood pressure and its symptoms; heart nutri-ent and cardiovascular support; relaxes the heart and heart arteries, prevents and reduces high blood pressure, prevents high cholesterol, palpitations, reduces organ stress; eases muscle tension, stress, anxiety, tension headaches, migraines, emotional upset, restlessness, insomnia; use long term to strengthen the nervous system and improve stress resistance; stimulates immune response by forcing a mild fever (then sweats it out); use for colds, coughs, flu, fever, mucus congestion, sore throat; can be gargled and used as a mouthwash, and used in enemas or baths; helps indigestion, gas, increases bile flow, eases mild gallbladder discomfort (but not gallstones); diuretic for kidney and urinary tract infections, water retention; use externally for itching skin conditions. *Antispasmodic, sedative, diuretic, astringent, nerve tonic, induces heat and perspiration.* The essential oil is not for internal use; flowers must be used fresh or will cause "narcotic intoxication"; safe in pregnancy and nursing; no side effects or known drug interactions.

Lobelia • *(Lobelia inflata)*

Also called Indian tobacco; used by Native Americans of the Northeast, who taught its uses to the colonists; use only in very small dose amounts, 5 drops is usually enough; muscle relaxant and expectorant for coughs and respiratory illnesses, sedates the coughing reflex and expels mucus; for cough, asthma, bronchitis, colds, flu, hay fever, pneumonia, tonsillitis, whooping cough, pleurisy; also for fever (causes sweating), vomiting, laxative, food poisoning; traditionally used for diphtheria, tetanus, and convulsions, to aid childbirth, and (in higher doses) to induce vomiting to cleanse the body of toxins; used externally as a counterirritant for sprains, strains, muscle injuries, bruises, venomous stings and bites, skin diseases; sometimes used in enemas instead of teas; an herbal Antabuse to stop smoking, binds to the nicotine receptors in the nervous system; take 5 to 15 drops before smoking and enough nausea will result to make smoking more unpleasant than quitting, also calms cravings; promotes a feeling of wellness and happiness, reduces stress and tension; nervous system depressant, muscle relaxant; cools the body. *Stimulant, antiasthmatic, antispasmodic, nerve tonic, emetic, sweat producing, expectorant.* Use in very small doses (maximum of 20 mg per day internally and externally) or nausea and vomiting result; extreme overdose can be dangerous or fatal; acts first as a stimulant then depressive to the autonomic nervous system, paralyzes the muscles (including breathing muscles) at extreme high dose; other side effects include sweating, tremors, diarrhea, confusion, rapid heartbeat; the traditional use to cause vomiting is not recommended; overdose is possible with external use, as herb is absorbed through the skin; avoid using lobelia if you have heart dis-ease, high blood pressure, sensitivity or allergy to tobacco, paralysis, seizures, shortness of breath, or are pregnant or breastfeeding; avoid use with psychiatric drugs; do not use if symptoms of shock are present.

Lomatium • *(Lomatium dissectum)*

Also called biscuit root or fern leaf biscuit root; used by Native Americans since precolonial times, effective in the 1917 flu epidemic; herb is only found wild and has not been cultivated, no one knows the population or whether it is endangered; antiviral and stimulating expectorant, used primarily for upper respiratory infections; reduces bacterial and viral replication and increases immune cells, clears sticky mucus quickly; has promise for today's serious chronic viral dis-eases; use for colds, flu, sinusitis, hay fever, allergies, asthma, pneumonia, bronchitis, tuberculosis, hepatitis C, HIV/AIDS, chronic fatigue (Epstein-Barr virus); mouthwash and gargle for sore throat, strep throat; douche for *Candida albicans* and vaginal infections; poultice or skin wash for rheumatism, muscle aches, backache, skin infections, wounds, boils, abscesses, bruises, dandruff; diluted tea as an eyewash for conjunctivitis; smoke for asthma and respiratory infections. *Antiviral, antibacterial, antimicrobial.* Possible side effects of nausea or full body rash; no known warnings or drug interactions.

Maitake Mushroom • *(Grifola frondosa)*

Immune modulator and adaptogen used in traditional Japanese and Chinese medicine, one of several therapeutic mushrooms, active ingredient is beta-D-glucan or D-fraction polysaccharide; adaptogen means it balances and regulates the functions and systems of the body; immune enhancer and balancer; normalizes blood pressure, cholesterol, triglycerides, phospholipids, blood sugar; normalizes liver function, endocrine system; promotes self-healing, and promotes adaptation to physical and emotional stress; increases resistance to cancer, limits or reverses tumor and cancer cell growth, helps prevent metastasis, enhances the benefits and lessens the side effects of chemotherapy treatment and anticancer drugs, particular use for breast, prostate, and colorectal cancers; used for immune dis-eases, chronic fatigue syndrome, HIV/AIDS, arthritis, bacterial infections, hepatitis, constipation, palsy, nerve pain. *Antifungal, anti-infective, antiviral, antitumor, anticancer, adaptogen.* Considered a food; possible side effects of indigestion or softened stool, rare possibility of allergy; may lower blood pressure or blood sugar; no direct drug interactions known.

Marijuana • *(Cannabis sativa)*
Herb (illegal since 1969 in the United States) that has high potential for safe, compassionate use; used legally and medically as an extract in the 1930s through 1940s; legal in the Netherlands today without problems. Controls nausea and vomiting, stimulates appetite and encourages weight gain, decreases inner-eye pressure, relieves pain; eases nerve pain and spasms in neurological dis-eases; use for weight loss in AIDS and cancer patients; prevents wasting dis-ease, anorexia nervosa; relaxes tremors and muscular spasms in multiple sclerosis and cerebral palsy; eases nerve pain in paraplegics and quadriplegics, amputation, phantom limb pain, spinal injury, fibromyalgia; eases migraine pain; reduces seizures;

reduces pressure and saves vision for glaucoma patients; reduces nausea and vomiting in cancer chemotherapy, radiation, and drug treatment; alleviates anxiety disorders, bipolar disorder, posttraumatic stress disorder, Tourette's syndrome, Alzheimer's dis-ease agitation, and depression; also for asthma, degenerative respiratory dis-eases, insomnia, sleep disorders, chronic pain, severe pain, PMS, Crohn's dis-ease, epilepsy, autoimmune dis-eases, arthritis, rheumatoid arthritis; muscle relaxant, laxative; compassionate use for chronic pain and pain of terminal illness. *Narcotic, analgesic, anticonvulsive.* Side effects last for one to four hours after smoking, up to a day after ingestion; reduces anxiety and pain, increases relaxation, intensifies senses, increases appetite, raises mood, increases talkativeness and laughter, increases self-worth, slightly reduces inhibitions without aggressiveness, slightly distorts time sense, temporary effects on short-term memory; no hallucinations, no hangover, no overdose deaths, nontoxic, safer than many medical drugs; may not work effectively for everyone; serious legal risk.

A
B
C
D
E
F
G
H
I
J
K
L
M
N
O
P
Q
R
S
T
U
V
W
X
Y
Z

Marshmallow • *(Althea officinalis)*

Not the sugary candy that goes by this name, and not the same as mallow; gastrointestinal and urinary tract soother and healer, heals inflamed and irritated mucous membranes, respiratory tissues and skin; promotes regeneration of tissues; use internally for gastritis, indigestion, digestive ulcers, gum dis-ease, mouth inflammation, hiatus hernia, water retention, urinary tract infections, cystitis, urinary gravel, kidney stones, arthritis; intestinal and bowel inflammation, diarrhea, irritable bowel syndrome, Crohn's dis-ease, colitis, hemorrhoids; respiratory tract uses for irritation and congestion; expectorant, thins mucus; use for colds, coughs, sore throat, whooping cough, bronchitis, and asthma; topical use for inflammatory skin conditions, dermatitis, chapped skin, wounds, bruises, swelling, burns, insect bites, abrasions, eczema, psoriasis, boils, abscesses, varicose ulcers; poison antidote, immune stimulant, detoxifier, and cleanser; use for muscular stiffness and pain; lowers blood sugar. *Anti-inflammatory, soothes, lubricates, diuretic, expectorant, laxative.* Generally regarded as safe and without side effects; may interfere with medications taken by mouth, use several hours before or after medications.

Maté • *See* Yerba Maté

Meadowsweet • *(Filipendula ulmaria, spiraea ulmaria)*
Herbal aspirin that is also an antacid, less strong than white willow bark, fewer side effects and digestive upsets than aspirin, contains salacin from which aspirin was derived; soothes the mucous membranes of the digestive tract, protects the stomach against irritation and bleeding; use for indigestion and acid stomach, nausea, peptic ulcer, heartburn, gastritis, esophageal burning; mild urinary antiseptic, diuretic; use for cystitis, water retention, bladder and kidney infections, rheumatism, arthritis, joint and muscle pains, sprains, aches and pains; also for diarrhea, especially in children, and for colds, coughs, flu, headaches, fever (induces sweating), wounds, insect stings, inflamed eyes (as an eyewash), blood dis-eases, anemia, chronic vaginitis, cervicitis, prostatitis; anti-inflammatory; for gastric ulcers or stomach acidity, use as a tea or dissolve the tincture in water to avoid irritation from the tincture alcohol. *Astringent, diuretic, antidiarrhea, anti-inflammatory, antacid.* Side effects include nausea, contact rash; tightens the lung airways, avoid if asthmatic; avoid if hypersensitive to aspirin

or sulfites; not for use in children with fever or infectious diseases because of Reye's syndrome; may lead to preterm labor in pregnancy; drug interactions with bismuth subsalicylate, ticlopidine, blood thinners, and narcotic sedatives—avoid taking with these medications.

Milk Thistle • *(Silymarin marianum)*

Can be used alone or with dandelion as a liver cleanser and healer; regenerates the liver, promotes new liver cell growth to replace damaged cells, protects the liver and kidneys from toxins, speeds up elimination of toxins from the body; used for hepatitis, cirrhosis, inflammatory liver conditions, gallbladder and gallstones; also used for liver damage from alcohol, chemicals, drugs, diseases, viruses, pollutants, toxins, and toxic plants; protects from the damage of some medical, antipsychotic, and chemotherapy drugs; also used for fat metabolism, diabetes, digestion, allergies, adrenal dis-eases, adrenal burnout; stimulates breast milk, brings on menses; possible use for prostate cancer, lung cancer, tumors, skin cancer. *Detoxifier, liver tonic, antioxidant, anti-inflammatory.* No significant side effects or warnings, safe in pregnancy and nursing; drug interactions are unclear.

Mistletoe • (Viscum album)

Sacred plant of the Druids, plant parasite, poisonous if ingested raw; used in Europe for cancer treatment but outlawed for use in or import into the United States; clinical trials are underway in the United States; use only with expert advice and supervision—***potentially very dangerous***; traditionally plant tincture was used for treatment of seizures and epilepsy, headaches, infertility, menopause, arthritis and rheumatism, nerve dis-eases such as chorea, high blood pressure, heart dis-ease and stroke, circulatory dis-eases, internal hemorrhages, heart tonic, urinary dis-eases, and respiratory dis-eases; in modern European use, it protects the DNA in white blood cells from damage by chemotherapy, radiation, and other cancer drug treatments, decreases side effects of standard cancer treatment, seems effective in killing cancer and tumor cells, and offers promise for increased survival and quality of life. *Anticancer, antitumor, cardiac depressant, nervine, antispasmodic, tonic, narcotic.* Raw mistletoe is poisonous, with potentially fatal side effects of vomiting, seizures, abnormal blood pressure, and reduced heart rate; medical injection side effects include swelling and soreness at injection site,

A
B
C
D
E
F
G
H
I
J
K
L
M
N
O
P
Q
R
S
T
U
V
W
X
Y
Z

headache, chills, fever, allergic reactions, and anaphylactic shock; research qualified European cancer centers if you are contemplating this treatment.

Motherwort • *(Leonurus cardiaca)*

Used primarily for "women's complaints," heart dis-ease, and to quiet the nervous system; heart strengthener and tonic; reduces palpitations, dilates the blood vessels, relaxes coronary arteries, increases blood flow to the heart, strengthens the heartbeat without increasing pulse rate, lowers blood pressure, and prevents blood clots; tonic for women's reproductive functions, hormone balancer; use for menopausal symptoms, hormonal migraines and headaches; regulates menstruation, PMS, cramps, prevents uterine infection; reduces stress in pregnancy, eases labor contractions, labor pain; prevents hemorrhage in labor and after delivery, speeds recovery after childbirth, may have contraceptive properties; quiets the nervous system; use for stress, depression, anxiety, nervousness, nervous disorders, fainting, neuralgia, pain of spinal dis-ease (disk dis-ease), insomnia, tremors, convulsions, pain relief; sedative, tranquilizer; also for fever with nervousness and delirium, liver dis-eases, improved vision, indigestion, stomach cramps, hyperthyroidism, goiter. *Antispasmodic, heart tonic, sedative, hormone balancer.* Side effects include diarrhea, stomach irritation, and photosensitivity; allergic reactions are possible; use only with expert advice in the following situations: pregnancy (may cause bleeding and miscarriage), clotting disorders, heart dis-ease, high blood pressure; may be habit forming when used long term for insomnia.

Mugwort • *(Artemisia vulgaris)*

Has many magical and protective uses but also medicinal, similar to common wormwood, once used as a beer flavoring; dried leaves are used as insect and moth repellent; as moxa used by acupuncturists, mugwort can turn a breech-positioned fetus to normal birth position and stimulate uterine contractions; can be used to induce abortion in early pregnancy; chew a fresh leaf for fatigue; place in shoes for sore feet; place dried herb in a dream pillow to induce dreams, increase dream intensity, cause lucid dreams, and improve dream recall, also for astral travel; use externally for abscesses and all pus-filled infections, fungal skin conditions (such as athlete's foot), skin tumors; stops bleeding, heals wounds and sores, clears toxins through the skin; use internally to bring on menses, reduce menstrual bleeding, for menopausal symptoms; aids infertility, eases and hastens prolonged childbirth, and expels retained placenta; can stop or reduce intensity of pending colds or flu, fever, strep throat and sore throat (also as a gargle), asthma; diuretic for cystitis and urinary tract infections, gout, rheumatism; digestive bitter, increases stomach acid and bile, decreases gas and bloating; laxative; and expels worms and parasites; calms the nervous system, seizures, convulsions, palsy dis-eases, brain disorders; euphoric and mild aphrodisiac, blood detoxifier, an antibacterial effective for staph, strep, *E. coli, Pseudomonas*, dysentery, and more. *Antifungal, antiseptic, anti-inflammatory, antibacterial, uterine stimulant, antioxidant, nerve tonic, bitter.* Possible side effects: contact allergy; can be toxic with overuse or large doses; not for use in pregnancy or while nursing; no listed drug interactions.

Mullein • *(Verbascum thapsus, Verbascum species)*
Brought to America from Europe, now known worldwide

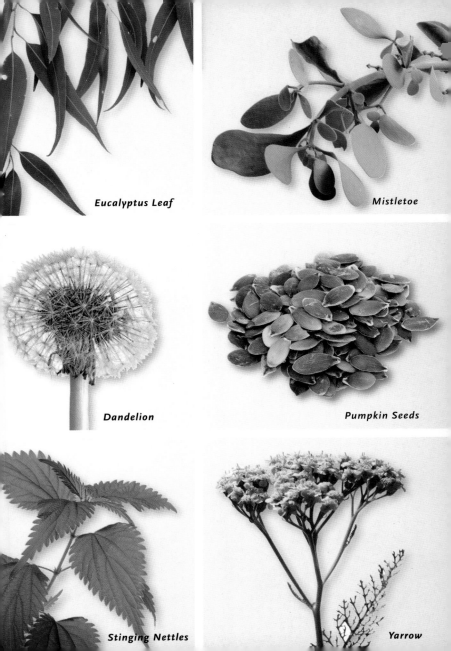

Eucalyptus Leaf

Mistletoe

Dandelion

Pumpkin Seeds

Stinging Nettles

Yarrow

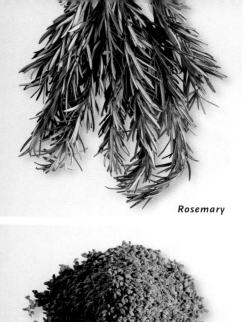

Rosemary

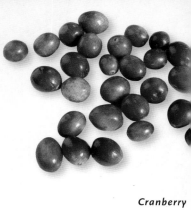

Cranberry

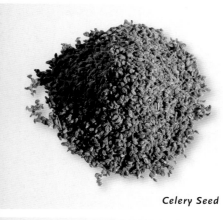

Celery Seed

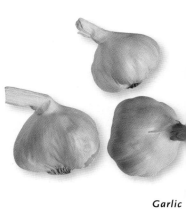

Garlic

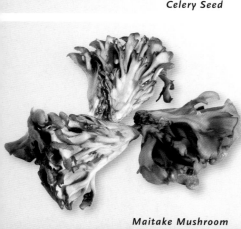

Maitake Mushroom

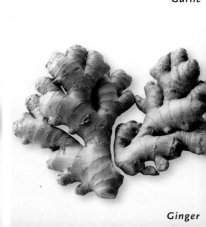

Ginger

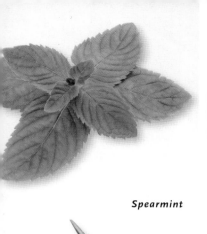

Spearmint

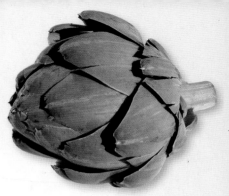

Artichoke Leaf

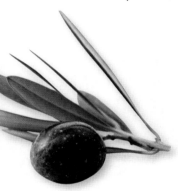

Olive Leaf

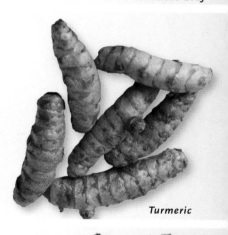

Turmeric

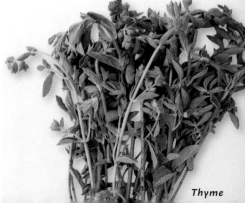

Cinnamon Bark

Thyme

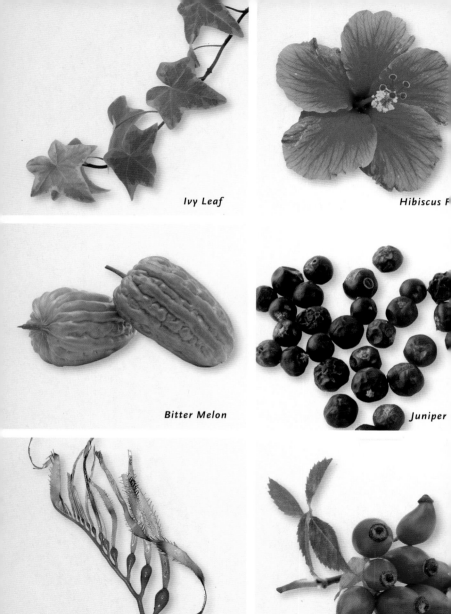

Ivy Leaf

Hibiscus F

Bitter Melon

Juniper

Kelp

Rose Hips

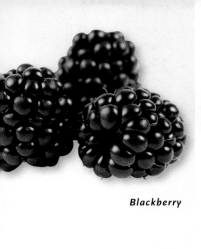

Blackberry

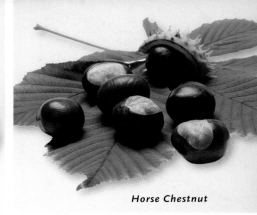

Horse Chestnut

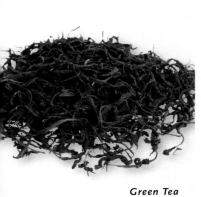

Green Tea

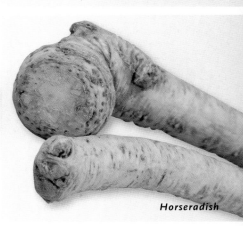

Horseradish

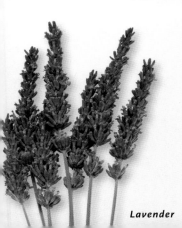

Lavender

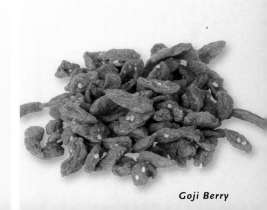

Goji Berry

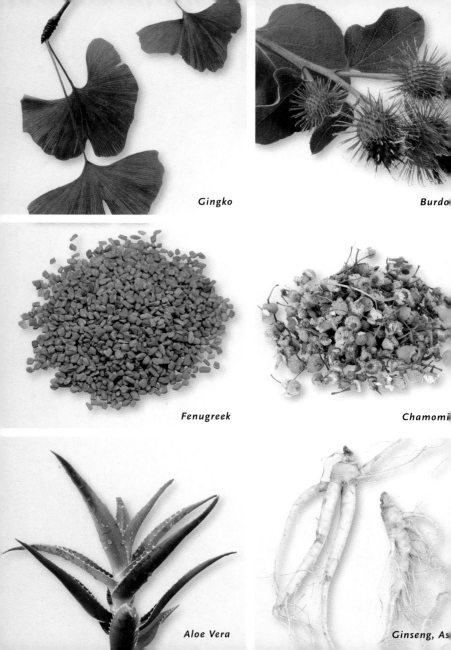

Gingko

Burdo

Fenugreek

Chamomi

Aloe Vera

Ginseng, As

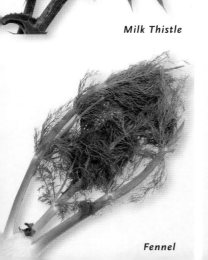
Plantain

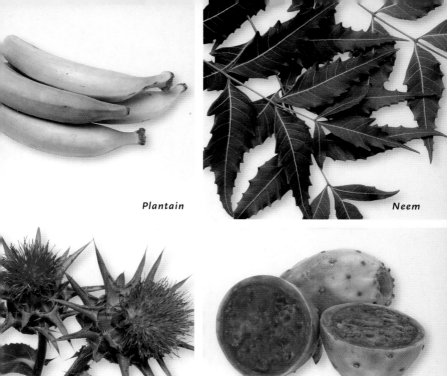
Neem

Milk Thistle

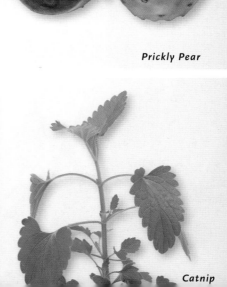
Prickly Pear

Fennel

Catnip

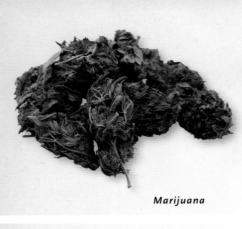
Marijuana

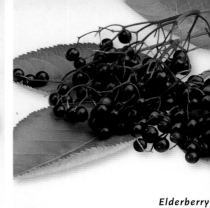
Elderberry

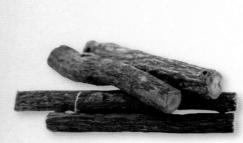
Licorice Root

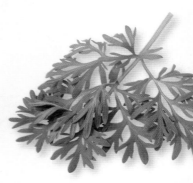
Wormwo

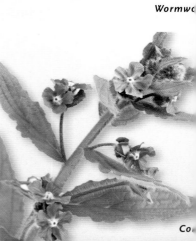
Sage

Co

primarily as a safe, effective herbal cough remedy; specific for bronchitis with hard cough and soreness; expectorant (thins mucus), promotes coughing up mucus, soothes irritation, relieves respiratory congestion for colds, flu, fever, sore throat, bronchitis, croup, emphysema, hay fever, whooping cough, tonsillitis; stops bleeding of lungs and bowels; traditional tuberculosis remedy; used to treat childhood infectious dis-eases such as measles and mumps; may be smoked like tobacco for respiratory irritation, cough, bronchitis, or asthma; also used as a glandular tonic, and for migraines, diarrhea, colic, cramps, convulsions, kidney dis-ease; circulatory dis-ease, heart dis-ease, palpitations, irregular heartbeat, angina; may have antitumor properties; external use for ringworm, burns, sunburn, frostbite, bruises, eczema, warts, boils, carbuncles, gum and mouth ulcers, toothache, varicose veins, hemorrhoids; mullein herb oil (not essential oil) is dropped in the ears for earaches. *Anti-inflammatory, antibiotic, antihistamine, expectorant, wound healer, sedative.* Considered safe, no known warnings or drug interactions; raw leaves may cause skin irritation.

Myrrh • *(Comminphora myrrha)*

Tree-resin gum used in incense making, as an aromatic, and insect repellent; indications here are for the capsules or alcohol tincture: do not use the essential oil internally; primarily known as a mouthwash (often with goldenseal) to heal gum dis-ease, gingivitis, pyorrhea, loosening teeth, mouth ulcers, tooth decay, and as a sore throat gargle for ulcerated throat, strep throat, thrush, tonsillitis, laryngitis; use externally as a liniment, healing salve for skin conditions and infections, swelling, wounds, abrasions, boils, carbuncles, aging skin, infected sores; use internally for respiratory dis-eases, mucus conditions, colds, asthma, bronchitis (internally and as a chest rub), sinusitis, coughs, expectorant (thins mucus) where there is low or no fever; brings on menses, stimulates uterus, corrects amenorrhea (lack of menstruation), may reduce fibroids, and used as a douche for vaginal infections, vaginitis, *Candida albicans*; useful in all pus conditions internal and external; important antifungal and antimicrobial, immune stimulant; increases production of white blood cells, promotes cell and tissue regeneration, inspires mental strength, mental clarity, and focus, relieves pain; digestive bitter for dyspepsia and gas, stomach ulcers; lowers blood sugar (diabetes), stimulates appetite; use for intestinal infections; expels worms and parasites; traditionally used for leprosy, syphilis, brucellosis, and glandular fever; increases circulation, stimulates spleen, lowers cholesterol, relieves chest pain from reduced circulation, prevents heart attacks and heart dis-ease, and prevents blood clots and strokes. *Antibacterial, anti-inflammatory, astringent, antiseptic, tonic, antacid, expectorant.* Works well in combination with echinacea or goldenseal; rare side effects: breathing difficulty, tightness in throat or chest, skin rash; not for use with high fever; avoid in pregnancy (uterine stimulant); may interact with diabetes drugs.

Neem • *(Azadirachta indica)*

India's ancient and modern all-healer, known since prehistoric times and still effective today; intrinsic to the culture and lifestyle of India with countless uses for every system of the body and countless nonhealing uses as well; used for indigestion, mucus congestion, allergic reactions, inflammation, diabetes, heart dis-ease (high cholesterol, high blood pressure, dilates blood vessels, prevents blood clots, and regulates heart arrhythmia), tumors and cancer, gum dis-ease and loose teeth, hemorrhoids, arthritis, skin care; douche for vaginal infections, placed in the vagina for contraception and protection from sexually transmitted infections, used at start of labor for easy delivery in childbirth, reduces childbirth bleeding; antiparasitic for scabies, head lice, and intestinal worms, insecticide; antimalaria, anticholera, leprosy treatment; blood tonic, blood cleanser, pain reliever, fever reducer, immune stimulator, diuretic; stops bleeding; used externally for inflamed skin, dry skin, boils, ulcers, sexually transmitted sores, wounds, swollen glands, hair loss, night blindness, conjunctivitis, earaches, deafness, athlete's foot, acne, psoriasis, eczema. *Antiviral, antibacterial, antifungal, antimicrobial, antiinflammatory, antispasmodic, antihistamine, and much more.* Extremely soothing internally and externally; too many uses to list; no known warnings or contraindications.

Nettles • *(Urtica dioca)*
Called stinging nettles for the stinging, irritating hairs on leaves and stems that disappear with cooking or drying; good cooked and eaten as a vegetable; use as antihistamine

for allergies and autoimmune reactions, pain reliever, antiasthmatic, anti-inflammatory, diuretic; reduces bleeding and lowers blood pressure; use for all respiratory dis-eases, allergies, excess mucus conditions, ulcerated mucous membranes, hay fever, asthma, pleurisy, bronchitis, pneumonia, colds and flu, coughs; diuretic for burning and difficult urination (cystitis, urinary tract infection), water retention dis-eases; aids weight loss, swollen prostate gland, arthritis, gout; reduces goiter, diarrhea and dysentery, fever; stops bleeding, including in pregnancy and after delivery, increases breast milk, reduces heavy menstrual bleeding, increases libido; general tonic, blood cleanser, poison antidote; use for anemia, skin, wounds, stings and bites, rashes, and hair loss and dandruff (as a hair rinse); reduces blood pressure, reduces heart rate, provides heart dis-ease support, increases circulation, dilates blood vessels, lowers blood sugar, aids digestion, gas, colic, lowers body temperature, and increases sweating. *Antihistamine, anti-inflammatory, diuretic, analgesic, antiasthmatic.* Possible side effects: skin rash, edema, gastric irritation, electrolyte imbalance; may increase the potency of diuretic drugs and heart medications.

Noni Juice • *(Morinda citrifolia)*

Tahitian and Hawaiian fruit juice, panacea and all-healer, whole body tonic and detoxifier, promotes cellular regeneration and healing; used for every organ and system of the body; pain reliever, antibacterial, immune enhancer, free-radical scavenger, digestive stimulant and laxative, wound healer; reduces inflammation, kills parasites and fungi, prevents cancer and tumor cells from forming and replicating; for arthritis, joint dis-ease, skin disorders, pus, boils, burns, broken-bone healing, eyes and vision, high blood pressure, high cholesterol, heart dis-ease, stroke, sprains, chronic fatigue, colds, ulcers, headaches and migraines, hair loss, viral dis-eases, digestive system, kidneys, ringworm, sinus, allergies, diarrhea and constipation, infections, menstrual cramps and irregularity, childbirth, gum dis-ease, fever, backache, sore throat, lymphatic system, intestinal worms, diabetes, circulatory system, intestinal dis-eases; promotes mental clarity and concentration, relieves depression, and increases physical stamina; the medical system denies these effects; the juice is sweetened to mask unpleasant taste and odor; dosage is usually 4 ounces of juice taken thirty minutes before breakfast, or

2 tablespoons of concentrate per day taken on an empty stomach (see packaging), the full dose is required for effectiveness. *Anti-inflammatory, antibacterial, antimicrobial, antioxidant, immune stimulant, antitumor, all-healer.* No known warnings or drug interactions; minor side effects of diarrhea, allergy, or rash, burping; claims to be safe in pregnancy.

Nopal • *See* Prickly Pear

Oatstraw • *(Avena sativa)*

Nutrient herb that can be used long term for people of all ages; high in vitamins and minerals, including calcium, magnesium, silica, vitamin-B complex, and vitamin A; helps hold calcium in the body; oatstraw, hawthorn berries, and nettles together make a delicious menopausal tea; provides a feeling of well-being and calm, cools the body, aids nervousness, nerve and nervous dis-orders, stress, exhaustion, burnout, depression, mental chatter, memory, mental clarity, balance, physical coordination, headaches, insomnia; tonic, hormone balancer for all ages, regulates menstrual cycles, PMS, cramps, menopausal symptoms, prevents osteoporosis, promotes bone density, bone growth, helps calcium deficiency; for pelvic inflammation, urinary infections (cystitis, kidney infection, kidney stones, gout), bedwetting; also for muscle spasms, efficient digestion, poor appetite, endocrine balance, rheumatism, arthritis, gallbladder, neuralgia, broken bones; heart dis-ease, reduces high cholesterol, improves circulation, stabilizes blood sugar for diabetes, provides support for addiction withdrawal; provides support for adrenals, liver, pancreas, thyroid, degenerative dis-eases, multiple sclerosis, lungs; loosens mucus in the lungs (colds, allergies, asthma); use in the bath for skin dis-eases, itchy dry skin, frostbite, wounds, boils, eczema, psoriasis, sore feet, joint pain, aches and pains, strengthens hair (use as hair rinse), weak nails, eye inflammation; good for pets and children's skin. *Antispasmodic, stimulant, nerve tonic, antidepressant, nutrient.* Safe in pregnancy and nursing, good for children; no side effects, warnings, or known drug interactions; no limit to amount or duration of use.

Olive Leaf • *(Oleae europaea)*

Used since ancient Egypt but receiving much modern attention; has the ability to inactivate viruses, bacteria, fungi, and parasites, and to regulate the heart and circulatory systems; used for immune system enhancement, chronic fatigue syndrome (Epstein-Barr virus), mononucleosis, HIV, herpes simplex 1 and 2, shingles, colds and flu, allergies, pneumonia, rheumatic fever, Lyme dis-ease, staph and strep infections, conjunctivitis, croup, meningitis, gonorrhea, malaria, dengue fever, tropical infections, *E. coli*, encephalitis; blood and intestinal parasites and worms, *Candida albicans* and other yeast, fungal, and protozoal infections; blood purifier and detoxifier; reduces high blood pressure, increases blood flow to the arteries, regulates heart rate, prevents blood clots, reduces high cholesterol, lowers high blood sugar (diabetes), and reduces uric acid (gout, rheumatism, heart dis-ease); also for achy joints, hepatitis A and B, severe diarrhea, food poisoning, blood poisoning, dental infections, urinary infections, skin infections and skin fungi, ear infections, intestinal muscle spasms; provides increased energy, sense of well-being. *Antiviral, antibacterial, antifungal, antiparasitic, antioxidant, astringent, antiseptic.* Side effects: detoxification may initiate a temporary die-off reaction for a few days or a week, with flulike symptoms, fatigue, diarrhea, aches, headache—reduce dose until the symptoms end

A
B
C
D
E
F
G
H
I
J
K
L
M
N
O
P
Q
R
S
T
U
V
W
X
Y
Z

if uncomfortable. Other possible side effects may include too-low blood pressure or blood sugar; may increase the effects of blood thinner, blood pressure, or diabetes drugs; should not be used with blood thinners.

Oregon Grape Root • *(Mahonia aquifolium, Berberis aquifolium)* A more-available substitute for goldenseal; can be used interchangeably with it; many uses, including indigestion, gastritis, abdominal bloating, nausea, irritable bowel syndrome, diarrhea and dysentery, reduced appetite, heartburn, arthritis, jaundice, fever, vaginitis (douche), green or yellow mucus discharge (indicating infection), children's infectious dis-eases, infections of all kinds, urinary infections; external and internal use for skin dis-eases, chronic inflammatory skin conditions, skin sores, psoriasis, itching skin, wet or dry skin rashes, boils, wounds; blood purifier, tonic, immune enhancer, anticancer; cleanses liver, gallbladder, and spleen; clears microbial dis-eases such as giardia, *Candida albicans*, viral diarrhea, and cholera; promising for diabetes treatment, lowers blood sugar. *Antibacterial, anti-inflammatory, antimicrobial, antifungal.* Not for long-term use, not for use in pregnancy or breastfeeding;

side effects include low blood pressure and heart rate, vomiting, lethargy, nosebleed, irritation of eyes, skin, or kidneys; avoid with tetracycline; some sources warn against use in liver dis-ease, while others suggest it for treating hepatitis B.

Osha • *(Ligusticum porteri)*

Sometimes called lovage or Porter's lovage; primarily for respiratory viral infections, coughs, and indigestion; use for colds, flu, fever, mucus conditions, nausea, sore throat, body aches, headaches, bronchitis, and chronic bronchitis, chronic cough, chronic sinus infections, colds or flu that won't go away, chronic or frequent viral infections and flu, chronic obstructive pulmonary dis-ease (COPD); promotes sweating and detoxification, suppresses coughing; expectorant (mucus thinner); antiseptic for the mucous membranes; helps childcare workers resist children's cold and flu infections, prevents secondary bacterial infections after viruses, helps prevent secondary infections for HIV/AIDS patients, helps prevent early colds and flu from becoming full-blown, enhances endurance and immunity; also for indigestion, appetite stimulation, toothache (poultice); relaxes smooth muscle tissue, eases painful or suppressed menstruation, retained placenta after childbirth; use for kidney dis-ease, urinary tract, and autoimmune dis-eases; inhibits bacterial infections. *Antibacterial, antispasmodic, antiviral, diuretic, expectorant, immune regulator.* Possible rare side effects include vomiting, dizziness, allergy usually caused by plant misidentification or contamination; may be liver or kidney toxic in long-term overdose; avoid in pregnancy and while breastfeeding; no known drug interactions.

Parsley • *(Petroselinum crispum)*
Food and culinary herb nutritionally higher in vitamin C than oranges, and high in vitamin A, amino acids, folic acid, chlorophyll, and more; improves potassium function in the body; use as a tonic and blood cleanser; strengthens the bladder, kidneys, spleen, gallbladder, stomach, and lungs; improves the elasticity and function of the blood vessels and improves blood flow to the pelvic organs; diuretic, dissolves kidney and gallstones, reduces blood pressure, LDL cholesterol, reduces homocysteine levels to lessen heart attack risk, neutralizes carcinogens and may be a cancer preventive; expectorant (thins

mucus) for coughs and lung congestion, brain and mental stimulant; digestive stimulant (colic, gas, indigestion, breath freshener, laxative); heals ear infections and may heal deafness; expels worms and parasites; pain reliever; use externally for insect bites and skin irritations, as a poultice for bruises, strains, sprains, and sciatica; use fresh in a vaginal suppository to bring on menses (also eaten or in tea), relieves water retention, contracts uterus after childbirth, increases breast milk. *Diuretic, expectorant, antioxidant, tonic, brings on menses.* Do not overuse or use long term; possible side effects: allergy, photosensitivity; avoid with kidney inflammation, nephritis, or in pregnancy; avoid with blood thinners.

Passion Flower • *(Passiflora incarnata)*

Similar to valerian but milder, can be used safely by children and the aged; soothing, pain reliever, mood stabilizer; calms the central nervous system, reduces restlessness, insomnia (including chronic insomnia), agitation, anxiety, worry, depression, headaches, migraine, nervousness, nervous tension, nervousness and stress, nervous stomach; use for nerve pain, neuralgia, shingles (for pain), diarrhea; antispasmodic action

A
B
C
D
E
F
G
H
I
J
K
L
M
N
O
P
Q
R
S
T
U
V
W
X
Y
Z

(muscle relaxant) for Parkinson's dis-ease, seizures, epilepsy, convulsions in children, menstrual cramps, colic pain, and all smooth-muscle spasms; antifungal, kills *Candida albicans* on contact (use in douche for vaginitis), tightens the uterus; as blood thinner, prevents blood clots; use with hawthorn for heart-failure symptoms of shortness of breath and inability to exercise; use topically for burns, cold sores, insect bites, razor burns, sunburn, scrapes, itching, hemorrhoids, eye inflammation and infections; prevents skin infections. *Antispasmodic, antiseptic, anti-infective, nerve tonic, antifungal, sedative.* Mild side effects may include rapid heartbeat, confusion, dizziness, drowsiness, nausea; do not use with anticoagulants (blood thinners), including aspirin and ibuprofen, or with sleeping pills or antidepressant herbs or drugs; avoid in pregnancy and while nursing; avoid for infants.

Pau D'arco • *(Tabebuia impetiginosa)*
South American all-healer and panacea tree herb comparable to India's neem tree, especially promising for immune diseases and all types of cancer; promotes resistance to viruses, germs, fungi, microbes; detoxifier, laxative; promotes red

blood cell production, replenishes all body organs and systems; balances blood sugar, reduces high blood pressure, prevents blood clots, heals the liver and heart, skin, lungs, joints, digestion; relieves pain, stimulates appetite, antidotes poisons and toxins; used for fevers, colds, coughs, flu, sinus, sore throat, allergies, hay fever, asthma, childhood dis-eases, infections, inflammation, digestive disorders, thyroid dis-ease, diverticulitis, varicose veins, menopausal symptoms, multiple sclerosis, lupus, AIDS, chronic fatigue syndrome, Parkinson's dis-ease, prostate dis-ease, yeast overruns, skin disorders; used for every possible dis-ease and symptom, internal and external. *Anti-inflammatory, antibacterial, diuretic, anticancer, antifungal, antiviral, antioxidant, antimicrobial, all-healer.* Has possible mild side effects of nausea, diarrhea, and blood thinning; no known drug interactions; safe for long-term use.

Pennyroyal • *(Mentha pulegium)*
Never take the essential oil internally, as even small amounts cause serious and potentially fatal liver and kidney toxicity, with symptoms of nausea, vomiting, abdominal pain, unusual fatigue, yellow skin or eyes, yellow stools, and little or no urine;

primary use of tea or tincture is to bring on menses as an abortifacient; do this only under supervision and advice of an expert herbalist, midwife, or medical doctor. *Antispasmodic, uterine stimulant, brings on menses*. Not for use with any medical condition, in a wanted pregnancy, while breastfeeding, or if you are taking any medications.

Peony Root • *(Paeonia suffruticosa, Paeonia officinalis)*
Traditional Chinese medicine remedy called mu dan, chi shao, or bai shao, depending on the tree peony variety; primary use is for women's menstrual issues, acts as a weak antiestrogen, female hormone balancer; regulates menstrual cycles; used for PMS, cramps and spasms, painful menses, heavy menstrual bleeding, high blood pressure in pregnancy, polycystic ovary dis-ease, female infertility; stimulates yet relaxes the uterus, increases blood flow to the uterus; also a blood tonic, stops bleeding or moves stagnant blood, clears blood congestion following traumatic injury, stops bleeding of wounds and nosebleeds; liver protector, healer and dis-ease preventive, used for hepatitis, cirrhosis, dialysis support (pain relief), high cholesterol (red peony, bai shao); emotional stabilizer,

helps clear long-held toxic emotions, increases mental function, aids dementia and Alzheimer's patients, prevents nightmares, epilepsy; reduces high blood pressure; relaxes spasms and cramps anywhere in the body, cramps from diabetes, chest pain; immune stimulant, pain reliever; reduces fever; traditionally worn as a necklace to prevent contracting contagious dis-eases; promotes clear, blemish-free skin, antiaging for men and women. *Antiseptic, liver tonic, antispasmodic, pain reliever, antioxidant, antiestrogenic.* Possible side effects include diarrhea (most frequent), indigestion, poor appetite, nausea, constipation, mouth ulcers; use in pregnancy only with expert advice; avoid with diarrhea from AIDS or cancer; may interact with the drug risperidone.

Peppermint • *(Mentha piperita)*

Primarily used and widely available as tea, found even in supermarkets; familiar flavoring for food, candy, toothpaste, and fragrance for shampoos, and more; grows wild in the garden; use the oil diluted only, externally only and with caution; uses below are for tea unless otherwise noted; best known for indigestion, nausea, diarrhea (catnip is more effective for diarrhea), colic, abdominal pain, stomach cramps, gas, bloating, irritable bowel syndrome; muscle relaxant; inhibits bacterial growth, induces burping; for headaches and migraines, dilute 1 drop of peppermint oil in 5 drops of salad oil, and rub 1 drop of this mixture on the forehead or temples, or undiluted on clothing near the head; calming, numbing, reduces anxiety, insomnia, depression; use for skin irritations (as a poultice or compress), herpes sores, hives, poison ivy, poison oak, insect stings; reduces cold symptoms; expectorant for coughs with phlegm, thins mucus; use for dry coughs, sore throat, sinusitis, PMS, menstrual cramps; improves bile flow, may break up gallstones; use for allergies. *Stimulant, antiseptic, analgesic, nerve tonic, antispasmodic, antiviral, antibacterial.* No known side effects with the herb; not for use with gastroesophageal reflux dis-ease (GERD), severe liver damage, gallbladder dis-ease, bile duct dis-ease; for infants, use highly diluted (good with chamomile); for colds, more effective when used with elderberry; peppermint antidotes the effects of some homeopathic remedies and should not be used during homeopathic treatment.

Perilla Oil • *(Perilla frutecens)*

Alternative to flaxseed oil or fish oil for omega-3 and omega-6 essential fatty acids, high in alpha-linolenic acid (ALA); takes as much as two or three months for effects; lowers the risk of heart dis-ease, stroke, and cancer; prevents blood clots, decreases cholesterol and blood pressure, protects the blood vessels and circulatory system; inhibits cancers of liver, breast, colon, kidney, and more; reduces inflammation and inflammatory conditions; use for arthritis, inflammatory bowel dis-ease (Crohn's dis-ease, ulcerative colitis, irritable bowel syndrome); heals and moisturizes the skin and regulates fat metabolism; used alone and in facial and skin products for eczema, psoriasis, cellulite, healthy hair, weight reduction; supports brain function, learning ability; reduces deterioration of aging, allergic reactions, water retention, and regulates the body's electrical energy conduction; cell protector. *Anti-inflammatory, antiseptic, vasoprotector, anticancer.* Use with expert advice in pregnancy, while breastfeeding, or for children; take at a different time from fiber; best avoided by those with clotting disorders, on blood thinners, including aspirin, or before surgery; may cause diarrhea.

Plantain • *(Plantago major)*

Common lawn weed that is almost an all-healer, also called snake weed; can be cooked like rice or ground into flour and used as a food. *See* Psyllium Seed for more uses; expectorant for respiratory congestion with mucus, stills the cough reflex, dry or tickling cough, asthma, bronchitis, hay fever, hoarseness, laryngitis, emphysema; cools the body to reduce fever; diuretic for water retention, bloating, cystitis, urinary bleeding, kidney stones and infections; neutralizes stomach acidity; use for indigestion, stomach ulcers, diarrhea, dysentery, gastritis, liver heat, irritable bowel syndrome, colitis, intestinal worms; stops bleeding internally and externally (some sources say only externally), reduces heavy menstrual bleeding, vomiting blood, bleeding hemorrhoids (poultice), bleeding from skin and wounds; many external skin uses: wounds and bruises, abrasions, cuts, bleeding skin ulcers, skin cancers, sores, insect bites, rashes, eczema, chronic dermatitis, shingles, tired sore feet, ringworm, eye inflammation, burns and scalds, poison ivy, snakebite, splinters (poultice); also used externally for mouth infections, thrush, toothache, earache (as eardrops); lowers cholesterol, lowers blood sugar; may be anticancer, especially for skin, breast, and colon cancers; causes aversion to tobacco (*see* Lobelia) and is being used in stop-smoking remedies. *Anti-inflammatory, antimicrobial, stops bleeding, expectorant, astringent, diuretic, cools the body.* Possible side effects: allergy, bloating, gas, diarrhea; no known warnings or drug interactions.

Pleurisy Root • *(Asclepias tuberosa)*
Also called butterfly weed or orange milkweed; used traditionally for pleurisy and typhoid fever; specific for the lungs and lung dis-eases; anti-inflammatory; thins mucus (expectorant), breaks fevers by sweating (diaphoretic), calms spasms, relieves pain and breathing difficulty; used for all situations of lung and chest congestion: pleurisy, bronchitis, pneumonia, viral infections, coughs, cold, flu, lung tonic; used internally and with enemas and hot baths to cleanse toxins and mucus from the body; other uses include colic, rheumatism, diarrhea, dysentery, indigestion; external use for wounds, warts, skin conditions, eczema, inflammations; has estrogenic effects, can bring on late menses, and may promote abortion. *Antispasmodic, diaphoretic, expectorant, tonic,*

anti-inflammatory. Toxic in overdose; side effects include diarrhea, nausea, vomiting, drowsiness, vision changes, irregular heartbeat, rash. Do not use in pregnancy or with hormone-sensitive cancers or conditions; not for those with weak pulse and cold skin, or those taking hormones or heartbeat-regulating medications.

Pomegranate Juice • *(Punica granatum)*

One of the first cultivated plants, pomegranates originated in Iran or Turkey and have been known since 4000 to 3000 BCE; high in vitamin C, folic acid, polyphenols, and (active ingredient) ellagic acid; juice is delicious but sweet and available in supermarkets; capsules have no calories or sugar and are safe for diabetics; has more antioxidant activity than green tea or red wine; prevents LDL cholesterol from attaching to artery walls as plaque, prevents atherosclerosis (high cholesterol, blocked arteries), high blood pressure; inhibits blood clots, reduces heart-attack risk; especially useful to prevent heart dis-ease in diabetics if used in sugar-free form because it has no effect (to raise or lower) blood sugar levels; important antioxidant (free-radical scavenger), prevents cellular and

DNA damage, inhibits cancer cell and tumor production, especially for breast and prostate cancers and leukemia; may inhibit HIV virus replication; reduces inflammation in the body, inhibits COX-1 and COX-2 enzymes that cause arthritis inflammation, protects cartilage and tissue from damage; reduces dental plaque, aids muscle recovery after workout, expels intestinal worms, aids indigestion; use as sore throat gargle; estrogenic effect for menopausal symptoms, prevents bone loss, hot flashes, depression; in pregnancy, may protect the developing brain of the fetus, prevents cerebral palsy, seizure disorders in the child. *Antioxidant, anti-inflammatory, antiviral, antibacterial, vasoprotector.* Caution with hypertension medications, otherwise no side effects or warnings.

Poria • *(Poria cocos)*

Called wu ling san or fu ling in traditional Chinese medicine; a mushroom-fungus plant used alone and in combination traditional Chinese medicine remedies; high in potassium, removes cold or hot dampness from the body; diuretic and expectorant to remove excess fluid (water retention) and mucus congestion from lungs and tissues; has immune-boosting properties, increases production of white blood cells, tones the internal organs (heart, spleen, kidneys, gastrointestinal tract, urinary tract), and prevents leukemia, tumor, and cancer cells from developing and spreading; tranquilizes and calms the mind for nervousness, restlessness, anxiety; use for insomnia, weakness, lack of energy, apathy, lassitude, amnesia; relaxes the muscles, organs, and mind; heals inflammatory skin conditions such as psoriasis, acne, dermatitis; improves the complexion; lowers blood sugar levels (diabetes); reduces stomach acid and acid indigestion, stops upper gastric bleeding, increases appetite; inhibits bacterial growth, including staph infections; also used for PMS, tinnitus, dizziness, diarrhea, chronic fatigue, anorexia nervosa, and palpitations; nourishes tissues and increases longevity. *Antibacterial, antioxidant, diuretic, expectorant, anti-inflammatory, anticancer, nerve tonic, immune enhancer.* Considered safe even for long-term use, with no side effects; use caution with diuretic drugs.

Prickly Pear • *(Opuntia ficus-indica, Opuntia species)*
Also called nopal or nopales; used as a food and available in juice, powder, capsules, concentrate, as well as in lotions, soaps,

and shampoos; high in amino acids; coats the gastrointestinal tract to prevent fat assimilation; protects from pollutants, drugs, and toxins; soothes ulcers and sore throats, acts as an antacid for indigestion; laxative (similar to psyllium); coating action also reduces blood sugar and insulin need in diabetics, lowers total and LDL cholesterol and raises HDL cholesterol, lowers triglycerides, improves circulation, and protects blood vessels from oxidative damage; prevents or reduces hangover when taken a few hours before alcohol; increases energy, endurance, and stamina; improves physical stress recovery, reduces fatigue; mood raiser; anti-inflammatory for arthritis, prostate enlargement, irritable bowel syndrome; strengthens the liver, urinary tract, and immune systems; use for immune disorders; inhibits tumors and cancer growth; aids weight loss, reduces appetite, slows digestion of carbohydrates; used externally for skin irritation. *Astringent, lubricant, antioxidant, anti-inflammatory.* Possible mild side effects: bloating, diarrhea, nausea, or headache; monitor blood sugar if diabetic; dried herb swells and can cause esophageal or intestinal obstruction; not for use in pregnancy or while breastfeeding.

Propolis • *(Bee Pollen, Royal Jelly)*

A nutrient rich in vitamins and minerals primarily used for immune enhancement; increases resistance to viral dis-eases, especially in changeable weather; protects against allergies (inhibits histamine reactions), colds and flu, viral infections, respiratory infections, bronchitis, nasal congestion, sinus infections, sore throat, mouth and stomach ulcers, liver dis-eases, gout, aging and cellular destruction; increases vitality and sense of well-being, cellular regeneration; helps fatigue, chronic fatigue, and immune disorders; may inhibit breast cancer, colon cancer, melanoma, and tumor growth; natural antibiotic, effective against staph infections (*Staphylococcus aureus*), inhibits bacterial growth, inhibits the bacteria that causes dental cavities, inhibits fungal growth; protects against and heals sunburn, acne, skin conditions, cuts and sores, shingles and herpes; normalizes high and low blood pressure, lowers cholesterol, prevents blood clots; supports the thyroid, glandular function, and treats glandular dis-eases. *Antibacterial, antifungal, antiviral, antimicrobial, anti-inflammatory, antioxidant, antihistamine, immune enhancer.* Can cause allergic reactions, skin rash, and mouth sores in some people; caution if allergic to pollens, sensitive to bee stings; avoid with asthma; drug interactions unknown.

Psyllium Seed • *(Plantago ovata, Plantago isphaghula)*

Seed husk of the plantain plant, used as a dietary fiber ingredient in foods, and as a bulk fiber laxative for constipation, alone and in many commercial preparations; works by swelling to a gelatin when water is added, to stimulate contraction of the bowel walls for elimination; mainly used for bowel regularity and for constipation, but the bulk fiber also resolves diarrhea and dysentery, dehydration from diarrhea, reduces bleeding of hemorrhoids, provides help for inflammatory bowel dis-eases such as ulcerative colitis, diverticulitis, irritable bowel syndrome; helps reduce cholesterol and high blood pressure, and stabilizes blood sugar levels in diabetes and hypoglycemia; used for obesity and overeating by creating a sense of being full and reducing fat absorption; used for ulcers, cystitis, rheumatism, coughs; externally for minor skin irritations, poison ivy and oak, insect stings. *Laxative, lubricant, anti-inflammatory.* Side effects include gas, indigestion, gagging; take with plenty of water to prevent choking

A
B
C
D
E
F
G
H
I
J
K
L
M
N
O
P
Q
R
S
T
U
V
W
X
Y
Z

and esophageal or bowel obstruction; avoid with narrowed bowel, bowel-obstructive conditions, or suspected appendicitis, or in pregnancy; take at a different time from medications and vitamins, to prevent decreased absorption.

Pumpkin Seed • *(Cucurbita pepo)*

Common garden pumpkin seeds, tasty snack found shelled in health food stores or easy to roast fresh; high in fiber, zinc, beta-carotene, and minerals; dose of whole or ground seed is 1 to 2 heaping teaspoons twice a day, about 10 grams total per day; increases male hormone production, helps benign prostatic hypertrophy (enlarged prostate), relieves difficult, burning urination but doesn't heal the problem; diuretic for irritable bladder, inflamed or blocked urethra, inflamed kidneys, cystitis, water retention, swollen ankles and knees, gout, rheumatism; reduces nausea, motion sickness, seasickness, fever, diarrhea; expels tapeworms and roundworms; high mineral content helps prevent osteoporosis (bone loss); strong anti-inflammatory for arthritis; lowers cholesterol, raises immune system response; high in fiber, reduces risk of some cancers, reduces depression, and promotes pain relief;

use externally for wounds, burns, chapped skin. *Antioxidant, anti-inflammatory, diuretic*. No known side effects, warnings, or drug interactions.

Queen Anne's Lace • *(Daucus carota)*

Also called wild carrot, a parsley family ancestor of the domestic carrot that smells like carrot; seeds are contraceptive; purchasing the seeds instead of wild-crafting (harvesting wild-growing plants) is recommended, as the plant closely resembles poison hemlock and fool's parsley, which are highly poisonous; to identify, Queen Anne's lace has a hairy stem; the poisonous look-alikes are smooth stemmed. Abortifacient, herbal "morning-after pill," written about by Hippocrates more than two thousand years ago; chew 1 teaspoon of seeds thoroughly, swallow, and wash down with juice or water; use daily starting just before ovulation and continuing for one week after ovulation; also can be taken within eight hours of unprotected sex, then followed by two more 1-teaspoon-per-day doses; the seeds may be made into a tincture (they are not pleasant tasting); works best for women with regular cycles, works least well for those coming off of the Pill; please note that all herbal contraception and abortion is unreliable—use at your own risk. Other uses for *seeds* include as aphrodisiac, nerve tonic, diuretic; brings on menses, prevents and dissolves kidney stones, treats gout, dropsy, hangovers, gastrointestinal discomfort, ulcers, chronic dysentery; expels worms; *flowers* lower blood sugar and may be a help for diabetes; *sap* is used for cough and congestion; *root* may be an anticancer and is delicious in soup; also expels worms and is diuretic for gout and dropsy; much more research is needed for this herb; be extremely careful in its identification and use. *Contraceptive, abortifacient, brings on menses, diuretic.* Side effects, warnings, and drug interactions are still unknown; not for use in a wanted pregnancy; caution with diabetes.

Raspberry Leaf • *(Rubus idaeus)*

Safe, traditional remedy for pregnancy and childbirth, available at any supermarket; drink two or three cups of warm tea per day throughout pregnancy to reduce morning sickness, prevent bleeding gums, reduce anemia and leg cramps, ease constipation, prevent uterine cramps, reduce miscarriage, relax and tone the uterine muscles, prepare uterus for childbirth, provide easy pregnancy and safe delivery, efficient contractions and shorter labor with less pain, easy expulsion of placenta, reduce bleeding and hemorrhaging after birth, less need for medical interference, promote baby's bone and skin development, promote healthy baby, provide essential nutrients, increase breast milk, help replace blood loss after giving birth, speed recovery after delivery, pelvic toner in pregnancy and after; also regulates the menstrual cycle, eases menstrual cramps, good menstrual remedy for girls in menarche, decreases menstrual flow; increases fertility in women and men; use externally as an astringent wash for wounds, ulcers, and skin irritations; use as a gargle for sore throats and internally for diarrhea (cold tea); brings down fever, eases spasms, eases intestinal inflammation and stomach complaints in children. *Astringent, tonic, antispasmodic, pregnancy regulator.* No known side effects or drug interactions; lowers blood sugar levels, so diabetics be aware; estrogenic, not for women with endometriosis, fibroid tumors, or reproductive system cancers; can interfere with absorption of some vitamins; take two hours before or after taking vitamins.

Red Clover • *(Trifolium pratense)*

Traditionally used as an expectorant and a mucus thinner, especially for children's colds and respiratory dis-eases,
cough, bronchitis, bronchial spasms, asthma, whooping
cough; may be smoked like tobacco for asthma; used internally and externally (especially with violet leaf) for chronic
skin infections and dis-eases, psoriasis, eczema, acne, boils,
rashes, athlete's foot, burns, sores, skin cancers, skin ulcers,
sexually transmitted sores, canker sores of the mouth; also
blood cleanser and purifier, diuretic; useful for gout; may be
anti-HIV, antidiabetes, and anticancer; contains isoflavones,
plant estrogens that may displace natural estrogens to prevent
or relieve estrogen-related symptoms; the literature is confusing here, as some says there is potential for cancer and heart
dis-ease prevention, while others say the opposite; possible
alternative to hormone replacement therapy in menopause,
with decrease of menopausal symptoms: reduces PMS, hot
flashes, breast tenderness; lowers LDL cholesterol, increases
HDL cholesterol, lowers triglycerides, promotes blood thinning, strengthens arteries, slows or prevents osteoporosis, and
prevents or reduces prostate enlargement and its symptoms

in men. *Antispasmodic, expectorant, sedative, blood purifier, antibacterial, anticancer.* No warnings for unfermented clover herb used short term; possible overdose effects are headache, nausea, rash, infertility (suspected in grazing animals, unconfirmed in humans); the "causes cancer" camp says not for use by those with estrogen-related conditions (endometriosis, uterine fibroids, breast cancer, prostate cancer), pregnancy, or for use with estrogenic drugs, tamoxifen, or blood thinners.

Red Root • *(Ceanothus americanus)*

Also called New Jersey tea because it was used as a beverage during the American Revolutionary War when English tea was unavailable; flowers were used by Native Americans as a soap for body, hair, and laundry; combines well with echinacea for medicinal use; increases the efficiency of lymphatic detoxification and waste removal, increases fluid circulation within tissues (interstitial), and stimulates the lymphatic system; astringent and stimulant to mucous membranes; decongests the lymphatic glands, liver, and spleen; expectorant; drains cysts and glands; used for swollen glands (swollen lymph nodes), enlarged adenoids, tonsillitis, pharyngitis (strep throat), sore throat, mumps, mononucleosis; also used for cysts of all kinds, including breast cysts, ovarian cysts, and testicular hydroceles; for all heavy mucus conditions, including chronic bronchitis, whooping cough, asthma, coughs, and lung disorders with shortness of breath; heals enlarged, swollen, inflamed, and congested liver or spleen; treats poor function of liver, stomach, and spleen; also stops bleeding, menstrual flooding and hemorrhage, nosebleeds, hemorrhoids, old ulcers, bleeding from coughing or vomiting; used for snakebite, fevers, dysentery, and as a sedative; used externally for toothache and mouth sores, sexually transmitted sores, and as a hair rinse. *Astringent, antispasmodic, expectorant, sedative.* No known side effects, warnings, or drug interactions.

Red Yeast Rice • *(Monascus purpureus)*

Rice fermented naturally with red yeast (*Monascus purpureus*), used in Chinese medicine since at least 800 CE; the active ingredient is mevinoline (mevinolinic acid), a natural form of the statin medical drug used for cholesterol reduction; works by inhibiting an enzyme that causes cholesterol production in the liver; lowers total and LDL cholesterol without affecting

HDL cholesterol; lowers triglyceride levels, increases blood circulation, decreases risk of heart attacks and strokes by preventing plaque formation on blood vessel walls; also used traditionally for diarrhea, indigestion, and to "invigorate the body." *Vasodilator, digestive, liver tonic.* Take with meals to reduce possible side effects of muscle or joint pain or tenderness, flulike symptoms, indigestion, heartburn, headache, dizziness, liver inflammation, or peripheral nerve damage; may be liver toxic in overdose; do not use in pregnancy or while breastfeeding, with liver dis-ease, for six weeks after major surgery or organ transplant, or during serious infection; do not use with cholesterol-lowering drugs.

Reishi Mushroom • *(Ganoderma lucidum)*

Also called ganoderma, probably the best known of many types of medicinal mushrooms; use 3 to 5 grams per day boiled into tea; fresh ganoderma may be more potent than dried; used in China as a preventive and cure for most dis-eases; strengthens the immune system, immune response, and immune cell formation; increases longevity; use for all immune deficiency dis-eases, also chronic fatigue syndrome, recovery from debility and surgery, fatigue, anorexia, altitude sickness, coughs, colds, flu, insomnia, stress, nervous and neurological dis-eases, allergies, dermatitis, headache, indigestion, asthma, rheumatism, arthritis, bronchitis, conjunctivitis, back pain, all pain; calmative, muscle relaxant; also for liver protection, liver dis-ease, liver failure, hepatitis, Alzheimer's dis-ease, HIV support, hypothyroidism, diabetes (lowers blood sugar levels); use for heart dis-ease, angina; increases circulation, lowers blood pressure, lowers triglycerides, prevents blood clots, reduces plaque buildup in arteries (atherosclerosis); antitumor and cancer preventive, said to change cancerous cells to benign, reduces radiation therapy and chemotherapy side effects (fatigue, nausea, vomiting, appetite loss, hair loss, sore throat, infections, bone marrow suppression, pain, all toxic effects), increases length and quality of life in terminal cancer patients. *Anticancer, antitumor, antiallergic, anti-inflammatory, antiviral, antifungal, antidiabetic.* Temporary detoxification die-off symptoms are possible: dizziness, itching, thirst, increased urination, diarrhea or constipation, soreness, pimples; these are considered normal; no toxicity or known drug interactions.

Rhodiola • *(Rhodiola rosea)*

Used in Tibet and Russia for a thousand years; also called golden root; benefits take from a few days to forty days for full effect; an adaptogen similar to Siberian ginseng; normalizes all mental and physical functions and systems, and protects the mind and body from damaging stress; increases oxygen and nutrient levels in the blood; increases resistance to chemical, biological, emotional, and physical stressors; increases resistance to dis-ease, both calms and stimulates; promotes calm energy, vitality, and well-being; mood stabilizer, antidepressant; increases endurance, athletic and work performance; enhances memory and learning, longevity; reduces fatigue, including fatigue due to aging; calms irritability, aids insomnia; promotes recovery from dis-ease and debility, tonic; immune regulator and enhancer; regulates blood sugar, protects from free-radical damage, prevents allergic reactions, destroys cancer cells, protects against the side effects of chemotherapy and radiation treatment; protects the heart, lowers high blood pressure, regulates heart rate, palpitations, angina, stress-induced cardiac damage; reduces inflammation in the body; also for altitude sickness, poor appetite, weight loss or gain, irregular menstruation, painful menstruation, vaginal infections, headaches, colds and flu, viruses, antiaging. *Adaptogen, anti-inflammatory, anticancer, antitumor, antioxidant, immune stimulant, tonic.* No side effects at normal dosage; overdose may cause insomnia, overstimulation, or rapid heartbeat; nontoxic; no known warnings or drug interactions.

Rooibos Tea • *(Aspalathus linearis)*

South African red tea or red bush tea; good-tasting beverage for infants, children, and adults, safe in pregnancy and while breastfeeding; can be drunk hot or cold and with or without milk, sugar, or honey; also used in cooking and baking; high in minerals, polyphenols, and superoxide dismutase (SOD); nontoxic and caffeine free; relaxes the central nervous system, heals insomnia, irritability, headache, stress, tension, anxiety, nervousness, depression, and high blood pressure; high in minerals for healthy teeth, bones, hair, skin; increases iron absorption; stops thirst, indigestion, cramps, colic in infants (mix with breast milk), nausea, heartburn, gas, allergies and allergic reactions, hay fever, asthma, ulcers, constipation; regulates appetite, exercise fatigue (as an electrolyte balancer or sports drink), hangovers; immune balancer, antiaging, heart and liver protector; kills cancer cells, reduces inflammations and infections, lowers cholesterol, prevents blood clots, fights free-radical damage; used externally, reduces skin irritation and inflammation for diaper rash, acne, eczema, skin rashes, sunburn, and skin disorders; soothing poultice for tired eyes. *Antispasmodic, antioxidant, anticancer, antimutagenic, antiviral, anti-inflammatory, immune regulator.* Very safe; no known warnings, side effects, or drug interactions.

Rose Hips • *(Rosa canina)*

The haws or fruit of the dog rose bush or other rose species, high in vitamins C, E, K, beta-carotene, pectin, and bioflavonoids; used as tea for a highly absorbable, though relatively low, source of vitamin C; 3 ounces of dried rose hips contain 1,700 mg of vitamin C (easily taken in 1 or 2 tablets from the health food store), but actually a higher amount of vitamin C than in citrus juice; rose hips are often included in vitamin C formulas; used as an herbal aspirin (though does not contain salicin) for many of the same things aspirin is used for; effective for osteoarthritis, as an anti-inflammatory and pain reliever; reduces joint stiffness and promotes flexibility, especially for hips and knees; tones the vascular system, reduces cholesterol and blood pressure, may help prevent heart disease; diuretic, relieves water retention, flushes the kidneys, prevents cystitis and urinary tract infection symptoms, dissolves urinary gravel and kidney stones; aids digestion, reduces hunger cravings for weight loss, eases constipation, diarrhea, and dysentery; balances intestinal flora, balances the acid-alkaline balance of the body; clears the bronchial passages of congestion and mucus; use for colds, flu, sore throat, allergies; cools the body to reduce fever; helps prevent infections, boosts the immune system and thymus function, protects from cancer, protects from environmental pollutants; blood cleanser; also for headaches, dizziness, nervous tension, mastitis, uterine cramps; reduces menstrual flow, vaginal discharge; calms the fetus in the womb; used in skin preparations and cosmetics to stimulate collagen growth, speed wound and bruise healing, and soothe skin irritations, rashes, burns, eczema, and aging skin. *Anti-inflammatory, antioxidant, astringent, diuretic.* Considered extremely safe, even in pregnancy and nursing; possible rare side effects:

headache, heartburn, nausea, or insomnia; no drug interactions or warnings.

Rosemary • *(Rosmarinus officinalis)*

An evergreen piney shrub that is actually of the mint family, used for food spice, flavoring, and a fragrance in soaps and cosmetics; do not use the essential oil internally, and if used on the skin, it must be diluted; uses here are for the herb (not the oil, unless specifically indicated) in tea, capsules, or tinctures; relaxes the muscles, including the smooth muscles of the digestive tract for indigestion, stomach cramps, menstrual cramps, colic; anticancer: studies show that eating rosemary herb reduces the incidence of skin, colon, lung, and breast cancers by half; used externally (dilute it), the oil protects the skin from cancer and from sun damage, inhibits skin tumor growth; stimulates the brain and nervous system, eases headaches; provides mild pain relief; memory enhancer, tonic, diuretic; use for rheumatism, gout; increases circulation; can be used externally as a hair rinse or mixed with shampoo (especially good with nettles) that lightens blonde hair and conditions all hair colors; promotes hair growth and stops hair loss. *Tonic, astringent, stimulant, anticancer, circulatory stimulant, diuretic, antispasmodic.* Safe in cooking or herb form, overuse can cause irritation and cramps; essential oil can cause autoimmune dis-eases, allergy, seizures, toxicity to stomach, kidneys, intestines; avoid in pregnancy except as a cooking herb; no known drug interactions.

Sage • *(Salvia officinalis)*

Also called common sage; most often used as a cooking and food spice; estrogenic for women's complaints of infertility, menopausal symptoms, hot flashes (drink cold); brings on menses, irregular menses, corrects lack of menses (amenorrhea), eases vaginitis (douche); promotes breast milk used hot, stops breast milk used cold; anti-inflammatory, antibacterial, and antihistamine used for all infections and inflammations; soothes mucous membranes, coughs, sore throat (when used as a a gargle), fever (promotes sweating when drunk hot), and ulcers; use for most lung and respiratory dis-eases, allergies, and tuberculosis; inhibits herpes virus, *E. coli*, staph and strep, dysentery, and more; use for digestion, gas, liver dis-eases; seeds can be used as a bulk laxative (like psyllium); lowers blood sugar, increases insulin effectiveness in diabetics, lowers blood pressure; increases mental and cognitive function used long term, possibly slows Alzheimer's dis-ease, reduces depression and anxiety; can be smoked as a legal hallucinogen (*Salvia divinorium*); external use for insect bites, fire ant bites, snakebites, mouth and gum sores (gargle), skin infections, vaginal infections (douche). *Anti-inflammatory, antibacterial, antihistamine, astringent, antispasmodic, antibiotic, estrogenic, antimicrobial.* Considered a safe herb but can be toxic in overdose and overuse with symptoms of warmth, rapid heartbeat, dizziness, or convulsions; not for use in pregnancy, avoid if epileptic; may increase the effects of hormone drugs, insulin, blood thinners, tuberculosis drugs, psychoactive drugs, echinacea, and other medications.

Sagebrush • *(Artemisia tridentata)*

The desert sage of the American Southwest, an aromatic herb high in camphor; not for cooking or internal use; used as a ceremonial herb for burning as an antibacterial and energetic cleanser, for smudging and in sweat lodges; repels insects and rodents from homes and food storage; first-aid disinfectant and cleansing wash for wounds and skin, insect bites, snake-bite, diaper rash, wet rashes; poultice for swelling, and as a hair rinse; smoke or steam used for colds, fever, headaches, digestion, and to relieve childbirth pain. *Antibacterial, antioxidant, astringent, anticancer, anti-inflammatory, antimicrobial.* This is an artemisia (wormwood/mugwort) family plant, not garden sage; not for use in pregnancy; external use only.

Saint-John's-Wort • *(Hypericum perforatum)*
Most studies find this herb more effective than tricyclic anti-depressants and with fewer side effects; however, it must be used for a long period of time to benefit; used for mild to moderate depression, anxiety, anxiety disorders, mental disorders, nervousness and nervous conditions, insomnia and sleep disorders, bedwetting, seasonal affective disorder (SAD), and recovery from brain inflammation dis-eases such as encephalitis; important as a sedative for nerve pain, body pain, back pain, fibromyalgia, and alcoholism (reduces alcohol cravings); used externally as oil for insect bites, wounds, burns, skin sores, earaches (including for children), hemorrhoids; said to expel evil spirits and psychic attachments from the body; used

for bacterial infections, including some resistant to antibiotics; also use for PMS, uterine cramps, irritability, food cravings, breast tenderness, menopausal symptoms, dysentery, diarrhea, intestinal worms, liver and gallbladder tonic; inhibits viral growth and has been used in HIV and AIDS studies, but studies were stopped because the herb interferes with the action of some HIV medical drugs; may induce abortion. *Anti-inflammatory, antiseptic, astringent, antibacterial, antiviral, sedative, nerve tonic.* Minor side effects: increased sensitivity to sunlight and sunburn, fatigue, skin rash, anxiety, dry mouth, dizziness, upset stomach, headache, or reduced sexual function; may increase or decrease effectiveness of medical drugs, including antidepressants, blood thinners, birth control pills, cyclosporin, HIV and cancer drugs; not for use in pregnancy or while breastfeeding.

Sarsaparilla • *(Smilax officinalis, Smilax species)*

South American rain forest plant that increases the effectiveness of other herbs and drugs, and is an all-system tonic, detoxifier, and purifier with immune-modulating properties; contains plant steroids called saponins but has no testosterone or steroid action in the body; used for immune and autoimmune dis-eases, cancer, high blood pressure, sexually transmitted infections, brain function, skin disorders, respiratory dis-eases and allergies, hormone regulation, liver protection, cellular regeneration; reduces high endotoxin levels to make this a primary remedy and possible cure for psoriasis, and effective for eczema, arthritis, ulcerative colitis; reduces excess androgens to treat acne, and useful for other skin dis-eases and wounds, burns, warts; other uses: aphrodisiac, sexual function, infertility, syphilis, herpes; decreases headaches, removes uric acid (rheumatism, gout, joint pain); expectorant for colds, coughs, flu, bronchitis, chronic bronchitis, allergies, fever (promotes sweating); enhances brain and cognitive function, memory, learning ability; useful for dementia, Alzheimer's dis-ease, senility, aging; also for pain relief, infections, appetite stimulant, PMS, menstrual disorders, digestion; increases urination; used in many herbal combinations to enhance general effectiveness; also for impotence remedies, detoxifiers, skin remedies, hormone regulators. *Diuretic, anticancer, antifungal, antibacterial, anti-inflammatory, antimutagenic, antioxidant, expectorant, immune regulator, hormone regulator.* No side effects with normal use; large doses may cause gastric or intestinal irritation; may theoretically decrease the effectiveness of sleeping pills and increase the effects of digoxin.

Sassafras • *(Sassafras albidum, Sassafras officinalis)*
Used today primarily as a beverage tea with delicious root beer flavor, offers zero carbohydrates for Atkin's Diet users, usually available in supermarket concentrates; formerly the largest export from the American colonies to Europe as beverage, flavoring agent, and medicinal; all sassafras products sold in the United States and Canada must be free of safrole, a component of sassafras believed to be liver toxic and a carcinogen; do not use sassafras oil or bark internally; do not use any sassafras product not marked "safrole free"; traditionally a blood thinner and spring tonic; induces sweating to break fevers, thins mucus (expectorant); used for bronchitis, colds, measles; diuretic for cystitis, gout, rheumatism, arthritis; painkiller, dental antiseptic, insect repellent, pituitary balancer, glandular regulator; used for syphilis; digestive bitter for appetite control, indigestion, colic, gas, stomach cramps,

stomach ulcers; used externally for poison oak, head lice, wounds and bruises, skin ulcers; stops bleeding, balances hormones, relieves menstrual obstruction; used as a tonic after childbirth. *Antiseptic, diuretic, tonic, expectorant, stimulant, pain relief.* Not for use in pregnancy and nursing without expert advice; do not ingest the oil: all available side-effect information is for the toxicity of the oil, with no known drug interactions or warnings for the safrole-free herb.

Saw Palmetto • *(Serenoa repens, Sabal serrulata)*

The most popular and effective herbal prostate treatment, affording relief usually within thirty days; often combined with pygeum; treats enlarged prostate gland in men (benign prostatic hyperplasia), and may prevent or treat prostate cancer; use for symptoms that include urinary frequency, especially at night, difficulty urinating, irritable bladder, bladder infections, sexual impotence, low libido, migraines, baldness; used in women for hirsutism (heavy facial and body hair), urinary tract infections, cystic breasts, polycystic ovary dis-ease (leading to menstrual problems and infertility), and for breast enhancement; diuretic and urinary antiseptic; also used for bronchitis, laryngitis, muscle spasms, digestive and intestinal discomfort; expectorant, appetite stimulant; stimulates low thyroid function. *Antiseptic, anti-inflammatory, diuretic, endocrine balancer, tonic.* Rare side effects include headache, digestive upset, dizziness, fatigue, constipation or diarrhea, nausea; may interfere with iron absorption; possible interaction with prostate treatment drugs and blood thinners; not for use by children.

Schisandra • *(Schisandra chinensis)*

Alternately spelled schizandra, called magnolia vine or wu-wei-zi in traditional Chinese medicine; has properties similar to ginseng but less strong; adaptogen to help physical and emotional stress response; improves general performance, increases energy, strength, and increases stamina, tones physical coordination and reflexes, reduces fatigue, reduces depression, aids memory, helps with anger control, aids cognitive function, promotes general wellness and vitality; protects the liver and liver function by activating an enzyme that produces glutathione, stimulates liver repair, normalizes liver function; used for hepatitis, chronic diarrhea, irritable bowel syndrome; also used as an immune modulator, kidney tonic, lung astringent, digestive (reduces overacidity); stimulates circulation, stimulates the central nervous system, increases disease resistance; used for colds, sore throat, dry coughs, fatigue and chronic fatigue, insomnia, night sweats, thirst, asthma, hay fever, wheezing, allergic skin reactions, headaches, dizziness, eye fatigue, visual acuity, palpitations. *Diuretic, adaptogen, astringent, antioxidant, antibacterial, stimulant, liver protective, cardiac tonic.* Possible side effects: indigestion, appetite loss, skin rash, heartburn, restlessness, insomnia, breathing difficulty; not used in early stages of cough or rash; do not use in pregnancy or while breastfeeding; one source says interacts with acetaminophen.

Sea Buckthorn Oil • *(Hippophae rhamnoides)*
Known in Europe, China, Russia, and ancient Greece; also called sea berry; nutritionally very high in essential fatty acids, beta-carotenes, and vitamins A, C, D, E, and K; used like vitamin E oil but more effective; for tissue regeneration, cellular protection, mucous membrane protection; accelerates healing for treatment-resistant ulcerative and inflammatory dis-eases:

canker sores, esophagitis, stomach ulcers, cervicitis, ulcerative colitis, erosive gastritis, acid reflux, Crohn's dis-ease, diverticulitis, chronic diarrhea; skin healing; heals the skin for acne, acne scars, rosacea, radiation damage, brown spots, stretch marks, scars, burns, wrinkles, wounds; promotes healthy hair; used alone and in cosmetics and skin preparations; also for sore throat, strep throat, infant anemia, pancreatic function, diabetes, tumors, dry mouth, arthritis, hepatitis, lung dis-eases; balances the endocrine system, heals digestion, enhances immunity, increases resistance to dis-ease; protects the circulatory system, inhibits plaque and reduces cholesterol, reduces blood pressure, protects blood vessel walls, reduces strokes and heart attacks. *Anti-inflammatory, antioxidant, anti-ulcer, anticancer, cellular protector, pain reliever.* No listed side effects, warnings, or drug interactions.

Self Heal • *(Prunella vulgaris)*

Also known as all heal or wound wort; can be eaten fresh in salads, soups, and cooking; a panacea all-healer used worldwide for virtually every illness and dis-ease; herbal antibiotic and antiseptic, anti-inflammatory, blood and liver cleanser;

stops bleeding, reduces blood pressure, and relieves pain; may be used internally and externally for all wounds and dis-eases; use as an eyewash for conjunctivitis and sties, mouthwash for gum dis-ease, gargle for sore throats, douche for vaginal infections, cream or poultice for external wounds and sores; use for fever, dizziness, diarrhea, internal and external bleeding, ulcers, liver weakness, jaundice, hepatitis, gout, heart weakness, coughs, colds, flu, allergic reactions; promising in recent research for cancer, AIDS, diabetes, Graves' dis-ease; used in a cream at the first sign of herpes (genital, cold sores, shingles), it lessens length and frequency of outbreaks; inhibits virus replication; immune system stimulant and enhancer; also used for bruises, sprains, burns, headaches, heavy menstruation, hemorrhoids, thrush, intestinal worms and parasites, gastritis, and much more. *Antibacterial, antiseptic, astringent, diuretic, antiviral, antimicrobial, antihistamine, anti-inflammatory, tonic.* No known side effects, warnings, or drug interactions; considered safe for all people and animals at all ages.

Sheep Sorrel • *(Rumex acetosella)*

Major ingredient in Essiac, a cancer-detoxifying herbal that includes sheep sorrel, turkey rhubarb, burdock root, and slippery elm; high in vitamin C but best supplemented with selenium 200 mcg per day; fresh leaves are high in oxalic acid, which is toxic in large doses, but cooking and processing should remove this; immune stimulant that increases white blood cell and T-cell production; blood cleanser and detoxifier for all body systems; eliminates toxins through the skin, strengthens the cell structure, regenerates tissue and skin, stops external and internal bleeding, increases blood flow to the abdomen, breaks fevers through sweating, protects from free-radical damage, relaxes the nervous system; primary interest is in its antiangiogenesis properties that reduce or eliminate blood flow to tumors and cancer cells; anticancer and cancer preventive; breaks down internal tumors, draws out tumors and growths when used externally for skin cancer, and also reduces side effects from chemotherapy, radiation, and drugs in medical cancer treatment; tonic and cleanser for the liver, promotes liver function, used for liver dis-eases, jaundice; diuretic and tonic for kidney and urinary tract, reduces water retention; use externally as a gargle for sore throat, mouth and gum ulcers; use as a poultice for all skin disorders and infections, boils, herpes sores, eczema, psoriasis, poison ivy and poison oak, hives, rashes, skin tumors, skin cancer; also for immune deficiency dis-eases, HIV/AIDS, chronic fatigue, muscle aches, fibromyalgia, diarrhea, pancreatic swelling, digestive dis-eases, hemorrhoids, bleeding ulcers, stomach hemorrhage, excessive menstrual bleeding, worms and parasites, appetite loss. *Antioxidant, astringent, antiseptic, antibacterial, antiviral, antitumor, anticancer, anti-inflammatory, diuretic, antiparasitic.* Not for use in pregnancy, while breast-feeding, or for children; should not be used with kidney stones, gout, varicose veins, rheumatism, endometriosis, arthritis, or hyperacidity; can lead to liver damage in extreme overdose; high-dose side effects include nausea, diarrhea, headache, and tingling tongue; do not use with laxative or diuretic drugs.

Shepherd's Purse • *(Capsella bursa-pastorius)*

Best herbal specific for stopping bleeding of all kinds, internally and externally; can be eaten as a salad green (mustard family) in spring, it resembles dandelion and grows as frequently; fresh herb is probably more potent than dried for medicinal use; use for hemorrhages of uterus, stomach, lungs, kidneys, wounds, nosebleeds; constricts blood vessels, lowers high blood pressure, contracts uterus; can be a permanent cure for heavy bleeding (flooding) in menopause, uterine bleeding, uterine cramps, fibroid tumors; used during and after childbirth to stop bleeding, vaginal infections (as a douche); urinary antiseptic for bleeding cystitis and kidney infections, blood or mucus in urine, urinary stones; diuretic for gout, water retention, rheumatism; poultice on feet or wrists is absorbed into the liver for jaundice; use poultice or compress for bleeding head wounds, external wounds, varicose veins, and as an eardrop for earaches; also internal use for diarrhea, dysentery, hemorrhoids, and bleeding colitis; may have anticancer effects. *Astringent, diuretic, anti-inflammatory, stops bleeding, uterine stimulant.* Do not use in pregnancy or with kidney stones; possible side effects: drowsiness, palpitations, high or low blood pressure, uterine contraction, skin irritation; may interact with heart or blood pressure medications or sedatives.

Skullcap • *(Scutellaria lateriflora)*

American and European skullcap variety; the Chinese variety has different uses; a mild calmative and antispasmodic, use for nervousness, irritability, insomnia, anxiety, depression, stress, nervous tension, and as a general tonic for the nervous system; traditionally used for convulsions, seizure disorders, chorea, and rabies treatment; also for neuralgia, muscle spasms, headaches and migraines, nerve pain, PMS, cramps, suppressed menstruation (to bring on menses), kidney detoxifier, hepatitis, infections, digestive stimulant (bitter), fever, and incessant coughing; a natural methadone used to reduce the symptoms of withdrawal for alcohol, barbiturates, tranquilizers, and opiates; currently being investigated for treating ADHD and nerve disorders. *Anti-inflammatory, antitoxic, antispasmodic, diuretic, sedative, nerve tonic.* Generally regarded as safe; not for use while pregnant (may induce miscarriage) or while breastfeeding; rare side effects of confusion, giddiness, stupor, twitching; no known drug interactions.

Slippery Elm Bark • *(Ulmus fulva, Ulmus species)*
Used as a finely ground powder, also called tree bark flour; highly nutritional, can be used by itself as a food for infants, debilitated adults, and pets, or added to oatmeal; as a tea or gruel, mix 1 tablespoon powder with cold water to make a paste, then add to 1 pint of boiling water, stir it in, let cool; also

used in capsules; soothing and slippery to relieve discomfort of entire gastrointestinal tract, stomach, intestines, esophagus, throat; heals all irritations, ulcers, and inflammations; use for diarrhea, gastritis, peptic ulcers, colitis, enteritis, bronchitis, bleeding lungs, pleurisy, arthritis, gout, coughs, cystitis, urinary tract irritations and infections; neutralizes excess stomach acid, clears mucus, cleanses, heals and strengthens, soothes; external skin salve or paste for all skin dis-eases and irritations, natural bandage for wounds, boils, ulcers, burns, abscesses, soothes vaginitis, gangrene, and psoriasis; as a poultice for swollen glands, toothache, rheumatism, and gout; in lozenges for sore throat and laryngitis; in an enema for intestinal worms and ulcerated colon; wet and insert in the cervix for a possible abortifacient. *Anti-inflammatory, mucilaginous, diuretic, expectorant, astringent, nutrient.* Totally safe with no warnings, side effects, drug interactions, or limit to amount used.

Spearmint • *(Mentha spicata)*

Member of the mint family closely related to peppermint and having similar but milder properties; good beverage tea and flavoring for food, candy, toothpaste, breath fresheners, chewing gum, and more; easily available in supermarkets; the major ingredient in the commercial Sleepy Time tea; easily grown in most gardens; calming, relaxing, refreshing, comforting; use for stomachaches and indigestion, headache, gas, hiccups, colic in babies, diarrhea, nausea, vomiting, colds, sore throat, stomach cramps, fever, insomnia; reduces androgen hormones in women to aid those with hirsutism (hairiness of face, breasts, or stomach); reduces smell of tobacco on the breath, whitens teeth; diuretic, used for cystitis, dissolves urinary gravel; eases menstrual cramps and reduces PMS; use externally for skin sores, insect bites, mouth and gum sores, dandruff, eczema, chapped hands, hemorrhoids, and as an astringent in the bath for oily skin; gentle enough for babies' and children's indigestion and colic; spearmint essential oil repels mosquitoes and mice, and is used in natural insecticides to repel and kill wasps, ants, and roaches. *Stimulant, antispasmodic, antigas, antiinflammatory.* Never ingest the essential oil; no known side effects or drug interactions with the herb; mints may antidote the effects of some homeopathic remedies.

Stevia • *(Stevia rebaudiana)*

Also called sugar leaf; South American plant that is three hundred times sweeter than sugar yet has no calories or carbohydrates; natural plant alternative to chemical sugar substitutes such as saccharin, cyclamates, and aspartame that are possible carcinogens; sold as a nutritional supplement, not as a food additive or sweetener; the FDA is foot-dragging on this one, possibly because of lobbying by the sugar industry; available in a variety of forms, used for sweetening, baking, and cooking; even comes in flavors, including chocolate; especially useful for diabetics because it does not increase blood sugar levels, may reduce them, and regulates the pancreas; useful for obesity, weight reduction, calorie and carbohydrate control, high blood pressure, limiting the sugar in children's diets, and reducing tooth decay; supports the production of beneficial bacteria in the intestines, helps those with *Candida albicans* (yeast overrun) on a sugar-free diet; supports liver function, reduces constipation; colon cleanser; may help indigestion and enhance immune function; used externally in South America as a wound healer. *Sweetener, antifungal, antibacterial, digestive, astringent, immune stimulant.* Nontoxic and no side effects; overdose results in bitter taste; no known drug interactions or credible warnings.

Stinging Nettles • *See* Nettles

Strawberry Leaf • *(Fragaria vesca)*
Leaf of the wild or domestic strawberry plant, food plant used as tea, fruit, jelly; high in iron and vitamin C, fruit contains salicylic acid (herbal aspirin); sold in the supermarket in tea bags; for indigestion and stomach soothing, diarrhea, chronic dysentery, appetite stimulant, spring tonic; diuretic for treating arthritis, rheumatism, gout, PMS, cystitis, urinary and kidney stones, migraines, and headaches; reduces fever; use as an antibacterial, uterine toner, liver cleanser; berries are antioxidant and possibly anticancer; juice was used traditionally to treat typhoid fever; external use for gum dis-ease, skin rashes and sores, frostbite, throat gargle, vaginitis douche; cosmetic use as a skin mask with oatmeal for oily skin, in commercial creams for wrinkles, freckles, sunburn, skin lightening, tooth whitener. *Astringent, diuretic, laxative, tonic, antioxidant, antibacterial, uterine toner.* No

side effects; no known warnings or drug interactions, no contraindication except allergy to strawberries.

Suma Root • *(Pfaffia paniculata)*

Brazilian ginseng, a panacea and all-healer; an adaptogen that normalizes and strengthens all body systems and functions, and helps the body adapt to stress; rejuvenates and stimulates, increases oxygen in the cells; tonic and detoxifier, calm energizer, pain relief, anti-inflammatory, endocrine and hormone balancer, antitumor and anticancer, cardiovascular and circulatory strengthener, central nervous system strengthener, rejuvenator and restorative after illness, antidepressant; increases resistance to dis-ease, enhances the immune system, lowers blood pressure and cholesterol, balances blood sugar, increases sexual potency and fertility, strengthens bones and muscles, increases mental clarity and memory; increases appetite, athletic performance, and stamina; used for asthma, arthritis, mononucleosis, chronic fatigue syndrome, AIDS, exhaustion, ulcers, anemia, sickle-cell anemia, diabetes, rheumatism, bronchitis, allergies; estrogenic for menopausal symptoms, PMS; rebalances after coming off birth control pills; external use for skin and hair; use for all cancers, leukemia, melanoma, lymphoma, tumors, and cancers of the liver, lung, and more; all-healer. *Adaptogen, tonic, antibacterial, anticancer, antitumor, antimutagenic, anti-inflammatory, immune enhancer.* Listed side effects are indigestion, nausea, stomach cramps; no known drug interactions; should not be used in pregnancy or with estrogen-sensitive cancers or conditions; inhaling the herb dust can cause an allergic, asthmatic reaction.

Tansy • *(Tanacetum vulgare)*

Herbal abortifacient and contraceptive, use the dried flowers and leaves only (or tincture made from them), **never the oil, which is toxic and can be fatal**; some bulk herb stores carry this, and the plant may be available in garden centers; be sure of identification, avoid tansy ragwort (*Senecio jacobace*), which is a fatal liver toxin; professional midwife or expert herbalist help is indicated when using this herb; to induce abortion, take 10 drops of tansy tincture in warm water every two hours (day and night) until bleeding begins; if the abortion fails, you must follow up with a medical abortion, because the herb may cause birth defects; as a contraceptive or early abortifacient, take a cup of tansy tea the evening before period is due—period should start by morning; or as a contraceptive, drink a cup of tansy tea once a day for the last five (not more than seven) days before menstruation is due (stop as soon as menstruation begins); expels intestinal worms, brings down fever, is a calmative for nervous upset; other uses: migraine, kidney weakness, indigestion, gas, cramps, colds; externally for scabies and impetigo, or as a liniment for sprains, gout, or rheumatism; none of the other uses justifies the risk: this is primarily an abortion herb. *Abortifacient/contraceptive, dewormer, digestive bitter, stimulant, tonic, brings on menses.* Side effects include nausea, vomiting, dilated pupils, stomach inflammation, weak or rapid pulse, coma—stop use immediately; use smallest dose possible for effect; don't combine with other herbs, don't take with vitamin C (may counteract tansy); not for those who bleed heavily, or have epilepsy, liver dis-ease, kidney dis-ease, or photosensitivity; use only with extreme caution and expert supervision.

Tart Cherry Juice • *See* Cherry Juice

Thyme • *(Thymus vulgaris)*

Culinary herb also known for its medicinal properties; an antiseptic traditionally burned in sickrooms to prevent contagion and used on surgical dressings; for respiratory mucus conditions and viruses, colds, flu, cough, sore throat, laryngitis, tonsillitis, colds, whooping cough, shortness of breath, bronchitis, asthma; use as a chest rub to break up mucus or as a sore throat gargle; breaks fevers by inducing sweating, relaxes the bronchial muscles; relieves indigestion, gas, colic, diarrhea; expels worms; use for gout, rheumatism, hangover, headaches, migraines; immune stimulant, circulatory stimulant, diuretic and antiseptic to the urinary tract; reduces high blood pressure, prevents seizures; brings on menses, eases cramps; used externally for cuts and wounds, swollen sores, warts, gum and mouth sores, athlete's foot, sciatica (poultice), in massage and bath oils, as a hair rinse and scalp massage for hair loss; considered to be antiaging. *Antiseptic, antispasmodic, antibacterial, astringent, antiseptic, tonic, antifungal, analgesic.* No known warnings or drug interactions, but best not used internally in pregnancy except as a food spice; do not ingest thyme oil.

True Unicorn Root • *(Aletris farinosa)*

Also called colic root or white colic root (several herbs are called "colic root," so compare by Latin names), often confused with false unicorn root (*Chamaelirium luteum*); whereas false unicorn root is used primarily for women's reproductive disorders, true unicorn is used mainly for poor digestion; digestive bitter, toner, and stimulant for stomach and digestive tract; use for inefficient digestion, indigestion, gas, colic in infants, anemia, diarrhea, dysentery, nervous stomach, lack of appetite; also for blood dis-eases, bronchitis, chronic tiredness, jaundice, and rheumatism; some sources mix true unicorn and false unicorn usage; a few sources include the following indications that are usually for false unicorn: threatened miscarriage, prolapsed uterus, vaginitis, and difficult menstruation. *Digestive bitter, antispasmodic, sedative.* Very little information available; no known side effects, warnings, or drug interactions; homeopathic form is available as *Aletris farinosa* (white colic root).

Turkey Rhubarb Root • *(Rheum palmatum)*

Known for its use as an ingredient in Essiac; usually used in combination with other herbs such as slippery elm to prevent cramping; not the rhubarb vegetable, only the root is used medicinally; used almost exclusively as a laxative and cleanser of the colon and gastrointestinal tract, thoroughly empties the bowel; used in small doses to relieve diarrhea, larger doses for constipation; ingredient in many bowel-cleansing formulas; also detoxifies the liver, gallbladder, and blood, and increases bile flow; encourages normal bowel function for those with chronic constipation; used for anal fissures, hemorrhoids; use before colonoscopy, after rectal surgery; stool softener, digestive bitter; use for indigestion, gastric disorders; expels worms, stimulates appetite, lowers blood sugar, may help diabetic neuropathy, kidney failure symptoms, stops internal bleeding, reduces inflammation internally and externally, heals inflamed mucous membranes, cools the body; stimulates menses, increases blood flow to the pelvic region; used externally for boils, wounds, skin diseases. *Astringent, antimicrobial, antibacterial, antibiotic, antiviral, anti-inflammatory, tonic.* Not for use with abdominal pain (possible appendicitis), intestinal obstruction, inflammatory intestinal dis-eases, history of kidney stones or gallstones, ulcers, colitis; for short-term use (eight to ten days maximum); may discolor urine, cause electrolyte imbalance, cause dependency; not for use in pregnancy, while nursing, or when taking cardiac drugs.

Turmeric • *(Curcuma longa)*

The yellow color in curry powder and mustard; used in Ayurvedic medicine and traditional Chinese medicine; an anti-inflammatory without side effects that is stronger than many medical drugs; liver protector that lowers cholesterol, prevents fat accumulation around the liver, stops biliousness after eating fatty foods, detoxifies, prevents liver dis-eases, jaundice, hepatitis, stimulates bile and gallbladder function; circulatory stimulant, improves blood flow, prevents blood clots, lowers blood pressure, reduces heart dis-ease; tones and protects the stomach, aids indigestion, gas, acidity, nausea, mouth irritations and sores, toothache; for inflammatory dis-eases, irritable bowel syndrome, ulcerative colitis, Crohn's dis-ease, arthritis, rheumatoid arthritis (COX-2 inhibitor); stops bleeding, helps prevent threatened miscarriage, reduces menstrual problems; immune enhancer; helps prevent cancer, stops cancer cell and tumor growth in breast, lung, colorectal, cervical, ovarian, prostate, and skin cancers; antiviral, antihistamine for allergies; external liniment for sprains, strains, bruises, bone fractures, swelling; antibiotic for skin ulcers, to disinfect newborns' navels, diaper rash, dermatitis, eczema, psoriasis, pimples, itching, herpes, leprosy, measles, chicken pox, snakebite, insect bites, ringworm, earache, eye inflammation, athlete's foot. *Antioxidant, anti-inflammatory, antibacterial, antibiotic, antiviral, antihistamine, anticancer.* Overdose side effects may include indigestion or nausea, and allergy from inhalation; not for use in pregnancy, or with ulcers, gallstones, or obstructed bile duct; do not use with blood thinner drugs, including aspirin.

Una De Gato • *See* Cat's Claw

Usnea • *(Usnea barbata, Usnea species)*
Plant combination of lichen and algae that resembles Spanish moss; herbal antibiotic considered stronger than penicillin for gram-positive bacterial dis-eases that don't respond to echinacea; antibiotic and antifungal that treats (gram-positive) *Streptococcus, Staphylococcus,* and *Mycobacterium,* but not gram-

negative bacteria such as *Salmonella* or *E. coli*; use for acute and chronic throat, lung, and respiratory infections with fever, staph infections, strep throat (pharyngitis), pleurisy, pneumonia, tuberculosis, bronchitis, sinusitis, colds and flu, coughs, also cystitis and digestive dis-eases; use for immune deficiency dis-eases, weakened immune system, autoimmune dis-eases, rheumatoid arthritis, lupus; muscle relaxant; use as douche or suppository for *Candida albicans, Trichomonas,* and *Chlamydia* (fungal and parasitic vaginal infections), treats cervical dysplasia; external use for abscesses, skin ulcers, burns, skin infections, skin fungi such as ringworm and athlete's foot; possible anticancer and antitumor uses. *Antibacterial, antifungal, antiparasitic, antibiotic, anticancer.* May be a skin irritant when used topically, may cause indigestion, otherwise no side effects or known drug interactions; not recommended in pregnancy, not recommended for more than three weeks of continuous use.

Uva Ursi • *(Arctostaphylos uva-ursi)*

Also called bearberry, used for more than a thousand years in China and Native America, called kinnikinnick when mixed with tobacco for smudging and pipe smoke; available over-the-counter for cystitis in Europe today; used almost exclusively for cystitis and urinary tract infections, kidney stones, pyelonephritis, urethritis; diuretic and urinary tract disinfectant, soothes the mucous membranes of the urinary tract, astringent (tightens tissues to reduce irritation and secretions), anti-inflammatory; other uses include external wash for sores, including sexually transmitted sores, and as a compress for back sprains and backache. *Antibacterial, astringent, diuretic, antimicrobial, anti-inflammatory, disinfectant.* The urine must be alkaline for best effect with this herb; avoid eating acid foods during treatment (tomatoes, citrus, pineapple, strawberry, kiwi), and take baking soda to alkalize the system; safe when used for short periods (less than a week) no more than five times a year; do not overdose; possible side effects include nausea, vomiting, insomnia, increased heart rate, skin rash, breathing problems, tightness in chest or throat, chest pain; turns urine green; not for use by pregnant or nursing women, children under twelve, or by those with liver dis-ease, kidney dis-ease, or high blood pressure; do not take with steroids or NSAID drugs (including ibuprofen).

Valerian Root • (*Valeriana officinalis*)

Used primarily for insomnia, stabilizes sleep patterns when used for several nights an hour before bedtime; use for weaning off of sleeping pills, antidepressants, and antianxiety drugs; sedative, reduces pain, eases anxiety and restlessness, eases nervous overstrain, traumatic stress, posttraumatic stress disorder; use as hot compresses for back pain (sciatica, disc dis-ease); antispasmodic, muscle relaxant; eases muscle spasms, headaches, migraines, gastrointestinal pain, digestive cramps, colitis, stomach ulcers; brings on menses; soothes brain and nervous system, neuralgia and nerve pain; anticonvulsive, epilepsy; eases heart palpitations, angina, and heart dis-ease; use externally for skin sores and acne. *Sedative, nerve tonic, antispasmodic, antidepressant.* Possible side effects include headaches, gastrointestinal symptoms, depression, nightmares, night terrors, and agitation; can become psychologically addictive; increases the effects of antianxiety and antidepressant drugs; not for long-term use.

Vervain • (*Verbena officinalis*)

Used in the last two weeks of pregnancy to stimulate labor;

Herb Listings

brings in breast milk after childbirth; medicinal for women's reproductive disorders when anxiety or melancholy are present; use with blue cohosh to expel uterine fibroids (reduces the side effects of the cohosh); use for menopause, menstrual cramps; brings on menses; also used to break intermittent fevers (causes sweating); expectorant (thins mucus), use for coughs, sore throat, bronchitis, asthma, pleurisy; internally and externally for headache, earache, bruises, neuralgia, rheumatism, gout, arthritis, hemorrhoids; external antidote for poison ivy; diuretic for edema and water retention; digestive bitter; use for liver and gallbladder, malaria, cystitis, indigestion, gastrointestinal spasms, bloating; expels intestinal worms; stops bleeding, reduces swelling; relaxant, pain relief; calms nervousness; use for insomnia, fatigue. *Anti-inflammatory, antispasmodic, astringent, diuretic, nerve tonic, sedative.* No side effects or drug interactions known; avoid in pregnancy until the last two weeks.

Violet Leaf • *(Viola odorata)*
Also called blue violet or sweet violet; its medicinal uses have been known and documented since 500 BCE; cleanser of

blood, liver, kidneys, and lungs; loosens mucus obstruction from all internal organs, cools conditions of heat in the body; used in teas and syrups for respiratory congestion and viruses with breathing difficulty, colds, flu, fevers, bronchitis, pleurisy, cough, chronic cough dis-eases, dry asthma, sore throat and mouth (gargle), swollen glands, sneezing, and children's dis-eases; also an effective expectorant, thins mucus, soothes mucous membranes, improves dis-ease resistance; softens and dissolves growths and tumors internally and externally for all cancers and precancerous conditions, skin cancer, cancer of mouth or tongue, throat cancer, colon cancer, tumors, reduces cancer pain; especially good used with red clover for cancerous conditions; healer for all skin conditions and swellings (use externally and internally), acne, abscesses, discolored bruises, infections, ulcers, pimples, boils, eczema, psoriasis, dermatitis, hemorrhoids; soothes digestive system; use for indigestion, nausea, constipation, stomach ulcers, liver congestion, jaundice, urinary infections, kidney infections, uterine and rectal prolapse, and rheumatism; reduces nervous tension, stress, insomnia, headaches, nervous disorders, epilepsy. *Anti-inflammatory, diuretic, expectorant, antiseptic, antispasmodic, anticancer, laxative.* Root may be emetic (causes vomiting) in large doses; NEVER use the oil internally; no known side effects or drug interactions.

Vitex • *See* Chaste Tree Berry

Watercress • *(Nasturtium officinalis)*
Used as a food and medicine since the ancient Greeks, called scurvy grass for its high vitamin C content, almost an all-healer; found in tea or as dried herb, rarely as a tincture or extract; cooking reduces or destroys effectiveness; can be grown in the garden; used for colds, stuffy nose, cough, lung congestion, sinusitis, hay fever, allergies, bronchitis, asthma; prevents the development of mouth, throat, and lung cancers and leukemia in smokers (must be chewed to have effect); high in iodine to stimulate a sluggish thyroid, heals goiter, balances the metabolism, reduces high cholesterol and high blood pressure, and stabilizes blood sugar (diabetes); blood purifier and spring tonic, increases appetite and also used for weight loss, anemia, indigestion, bad breath, constipation, debility, lethargy; increases stamina, eases headaches, reduces

stress and pain, joint and back stiffness, night vision; stops hemorrhaging, bleeding gums; strengthens liver, spleen, heart, circulatory system, glandular system, skeletal system, nervous system, brain function, memory; diuretic, kidney and gallstones, enlarged prostate, swollen feet and ankles; brings on menses, increases breast milk; external use for skin: acne, whiteheads, blackheads, scabies, eczema, fades freckles, healthy hair. *Antioxidant, digestive stimulant, anticancer, antibiotic, antibacterial, diuretic, expectorant.* Not for children under four years, or people with stomach ulcers or nephritis; may cause indigestion; no known drug interactions.

White Oak Bark • *(Quercus alba)*

Astringent and antiseptic, primarily used to stop bleeding and shrink tissues; antidote for drug allergies and chemotherapy side effects; stops diarrhea, dysentery, expels intestinal worms and parasites; stops internal or external bleeding, excessive menstrual flow and hemorrhage, nosebleeds, bleeding hemorrhoids, bleeding wounds, bleeding of lungs, bowels, stomach, and spitting of blood, blood in urine; also for fever, sinus congestion; prevents and stops bacterial infections; increases urine flow to wash out cystitis/bladder infections, kidney stones, and gallstones, ulcerated bladder; use for liver, jaundice, spleen, sexually trasmitted infections, vomiting, tumors, strep throat, ulcers, varicose veins (internally and as a poultice); use in a hot (but not scalding) water douche for vaginal infections and uterine dis-eases; in a hot-water enema for parasitic worms and hemorrhoids; use externally to stop wound bleeding, and for burns, stings, mouth sores, goiter, herpes sores, hemorrhoids, tumors, and as a liniment. *Astringent, antiseptic, antibacterial, anti-inflammatory, stops bleeding.* Not for long-term use. No known side effects; may inhibit the absorption of antacid medications.

White Willow Bark • *(Salix alba)*

Herbal aspirin, the herb from which aspirin was derived and developed, the active chemical ingredient is salicin; known since 500 BCE and earlier; slower-acting but longer-lasting effects with less digestive upset than aspirin; may be more effective than aspirin because of other compounds in the herb; used as for aspirin for all inflammatory conditions and pain relief: fever, migraine, headache, low back pain, nerve pain,

muscle pain, chills, wounds, toothache, osteoarthritis, rheumatoid arthritis, bursitis, tendonitis, tonsillitis, mouth and gum
sores, menstrual cramps, flu, dysentery, aches and pains, autoimmune inflammation, kidney and bladder irritation; prevents
pain messages from reaching the brain; prevents blood clots.
Anti-inflammatory, analgesic, astringent, antioxidant, antisep-
tic, immune enhancer, antiprostaglandin, tonic. Side effects may
include mild indigestion, skin rash, nausea, vomiting, and tinnitus; not for use by children under sixteen years old with fever
because of the risk of Reye's syndrome, or for use in pregnancy;
avoid if allergic to aspirin, or with gastritis, asthma, diabetes,
gout, ulcers, bleeding disorders, or when taking blood-thinning
drugs; drug contraindications are the same as for aspirin; check
before using willow with medications.

Wild Cherry • *(Prunus serotina, Prunus virginiana)*
The first cough syrup, known in Europe and Native America,
made with ground wild cherry bark, honey, and water, and
often combined with other herbs; only the bark is safe to use;
stops spasms in the smooth muscles lining the bronchioles,
sedates the coughing reflex, increases respiration, loosens

mucus and congestion in chest and throat; for irritating and persistent coughs, dry coughs, nervous cough, bronchitis, whooping cough, asthma, allergic coughs, aftereffects of asthma and allergy attacks, chronic obstructive pulmonary dis-ease (COPD); also used for chronic diarrhea and dysentery (cold tea), indigestion (a digestive bitter); stimulates digestion and appetite, relieves nervous indigestion; pain relief, cancer pain, sedative, insomnia treatment (contains a high level of melatonin); tonic, blood purifier, immune enhancer, lung stimulant, anticancer; wash for eye inflammation, poultice for sores and abscesses, enema for hemorrhoids; eases labor pains. *Astringent, sedative, antispasmodic, anticancer, digestive bitter, expectorant.* Can cause drowsiness; extreme overdose can theoretically result in cyanide poisoning; no known drug interactions; some sources list as not for use in pregnancy or while breastfeeding.

Wild Oregano Oil • *(Origanum vulgare)*

This is not the cooking herb but a highly potent all-healing essential oil; comes in prepared capsules or as *oil that must be diluted* to be safe; dosage: start with 1 or 2 drops daily in a glass of juice or water, increase gradually to 1 drop three or four times per day in a glass of juice or water; use for two weeks, stop for two weeks; honey can be added for taste; for topical use, dilute 1 drop of oil to 1 teaspoon of olive or salad oil; **Never use the undiluted oil**; potent antibiotic possibly stronger than penicillin or other antibiotic drugs and useful for drug-resistant germ strains; contains fifty antibacterial compounds against such germs as *Staphylococcus aureus, E. coli, Pseudomonas,* and others; antimicrobial for use against yeasts, fungi, molds, amoebas, protozoa; a proportion of 1:4,000 sterilizes unclean water; used for every kind of bacterial, viral, and parasitic dis-ease condition, including *Candida albicans,* giardia, chronic fatigue syndrome, fibromyalgia, food poisoning, pneumonia, asthma, arthritis, allergies and hay fever, irritable bowel syndrome, stomach disorders, gas, bladder infections, diarrhea and constipation, toothache, ear infections, cough, flu, rheumatism, muscle aches, varicose veins, athlete's foot, respiratory infections, sore throat, tonsillitis, sinusitis, colds, and irregular menses; external use for skin infections, itching, insect bites, diaper rash, acne, herpes, rosacea, ringworm, rash, psoriasis, eczema, warts; gargle in water for gums, mouth, teeth, and throat; use in a hair rinse for dandruff, scalp sores, hair loss; also lowers blood pressure. *Anti-inflammatory, antifungal, antiparasitic, antibacterial, antiseptic, antibiotic, antioxidant, antimicrobial.* No known side effects, no list of warnings except to use diluted only.

Wild Yam • *(Discorea villosa)*

Nonestrogenic herbal alternative to hormone replacement therapy drugs; theorized to contain hormone (progesterone) precursors but not actual hormones—science doesn't know how it works; best known for reducing menopausal symptoms of vaginal dryness, osteoporosis, hot flashes, night sweats, involuntary urination, urinary frequency, low sex drive, menopausal headaches and migraines, mood changes, memory loss, weight gain, as well as menstrual cramps and PMS; used in younger women for PMS, menstrual irregularity, cramps, spasms, cystitis, endometriosis, childbirth pain, after-pains, can be used to prevent miscarriage, for fertility and for contraception; use for all "female troubles"; increases energy and stamina, lowers cholesterol; use for cancer and heart dis-ease prevention; also a hormonal precursor to cortisone for use with inflammatory conditions: asthma, arthritis, colic, inflammatory bowel dis-eases such as irritable bowel syndrome, Crohn's dis-ease, diverticulitis, colitis, gastritis, gallbladder dis-ease, chronic diarrhea, boils, and abscesses. *Anti-inflammatory, antispasmodic, glandular, hormone precursor.* Considered safe to use long term with no significant side effects; usually used as a vaginal cream or liquid tincture; overdose may cause nausea, vomiting, or diarrhea, possible allergic skin rash; use in pregnancy or while nursing only with expert advice; avoid with liver dis-ease and hormone-sensitive cancers or conditions; may interfere with the effectiveness of hormone replacement therapy or birth control medications.

Wintergreen • *(Gaultheria procumbens)*

Active ingredient is methyl salicylate; only the dried herb (in capsules, tea, or tincture) is safe for internal use; wintergreen oil is toxic and only for external use as poultice, compress, or liniment; external use for rheumatism, joint pain, muscle pain, arthritis, lumbago, sciatica, back pain, boils, sores, swelling; gargle tea for sore throats, chew root for prevention of tooth decay, use in a steam tent to break up respiratory mucus congestion; traditional internal use as herb tea or tincture *(not the oil)* for colds, flu, headaches, fever, chronic mucus conditions; also used for indigestion, gas, colic; as a diuretic, use for cystitis, kidney infections; brings on menses, promotes menstrual flow, stimulates breast milk; also can be used in tea or tinctures for heart stimulant and tonic, to improve respiration, and open bowel obstructions. *Antiseptic, anti-inflammatory, diuretic, tonic, astringent, stimulant, aromatic.* Use herb in small doses; may be a contact allergen; do not use with tinnitus or if allergic to aspirin; **never use the oil internally**—it is highly poisonous; many better and safer herbs are available.

Witch Hazel • *(Hamamelis virginiana)*

This is the herb (leaf and bark); the liniment is for external use only; be aware of the homeopathic remedy as well; tones and contracts the veins and internal organs, and stops internal and external bleeding, very useful for menopausal difficulties; excellent internally and as a poultice for varicose veins, burst veins, spider veins, painful heavy legs, phlebitis (blood clots), hemorrhoids; stops menstrual flooding, excessive menstruation, pelvic blood congestion, menstrual cramps, uterine or abdominal prolapse, aids recovery after abortion or miscarriage, douche for vaginitis, compress for sore nipples; used for all passive hemorrhages internal and external in all organs, bleeding lung dis-eases, intestinal bleeding, nose-bleeds; also used for diarrhea, dysentery, colitis, mucus conditions, sinus and nasal congestion, headaches, pain relief; as a gargle for sore throats, tonsillitis, laryngitis, and gum disease; used traditionally for tuberculosis (lung bleeding) and sexually transmitted sores; external use as a liniment for sore muscles, sprains, swelling, bruises, external tumors, and as first aid for inflamed and irritated skin tissue, cuts, burns, scalds, insect bites, fire ant bites, inflamed eyelids, bedsores, acne, blemishes, poison ivy, and poison oak; cosmetic use for oily skin, also tightens (astringent), and tones. *Astringent, tonic, sedative, anti-inflammatory, stops bleeding.* Possible side effects of skin or stomach irritation, cramps, nausea, vomiting, or constipation; may interfere with some medical drugs; avoid in pregnancy.

Wood Betony • *(Stachys officinalis)*

Remedy for all maladies of the head: headache, hypertension headache, nervous stress headache, sinus headache, migraine, neuralgia, convulsions, toothache; stops bleeding of mouth, nose, or lungs; tonic for the nervous system, calms, relaxes, reduces anxiety and stress, nervous disorders, nervous debility; also treats respiratory tract inflammation and infections, colds, flu, cough, sinusitis, asthma, bronchitis, wheezing, shortness of breath; diuretic for gout, rheumatism, kidneys and bladder, edema, water retention; detoxifies the liver and spleen, jaundice; also for diarrhea, heartburn, varicose veins, intestinal worms, hernia, rheumatoid arthritis, increasing breast milk; external use for skin wounds, bruises, infected sores and ulcers, shingles, boils, sprains; usa as a poultice to draw out splinters. *Astringent, diuretic, bitter, nerve tonic.* May cause indigestion or vomiting with overdose; no known warnings or drug interactions.

Wormwood • *(Artemesia absinthium)*

Herb related to mugwort and sagebrush, primarily used to clear worms and parasites from the body; best used in professionally designed combinations (usually with black walnut hulls and other herbs); best used with expert direction and supervision; look for "thujone free" formulas, and **never use the oil internally**; expels worms, especially roundworm and threadworm; helps inefficient digestion, poor appetite, poor circulation; liver and gallbladder tonic; use for gas, bloating, indigestion after meals; increases nutrient absorption, increases stomach acid and bile flow; use for jaundice, debility after illness, depression, nervousness and nervous disorders; counters effects of poisoning from hemlock and other toxic plants, possible help for anorexia nervosa; used by midwives to speed childbirth and expel the placenta; external use for bruises, bites, compress for strains and sprains, muscle-relaxing liniment. *Anti-inflammatory, antispasmodic, antiseptic, antitumor, bitter tonic.* Safe only in small doses and only for short-term use, poisonous in large quantities; side effects include seizures, insomnia, nightmares, nerve disorders, trembling, stupor, headaches, brain damage; can be habit forming; not for use in pregnancy or while breastfeeding, not for infants or children; rated "dangerous" in the United States and "slightly dangerous" in most other countries.

Yarrow • *(Achillea millefolium)*

Contains salicylic acid (chemically similar to aspirin); used primarily to stop bleeding, reduce mucus, and as a tonic for blood, circulatory system, stomach, liver, urinary tract, glandular system, and uterus; external topical use for wounds, cuts, abrasions, poison ivy, poison oak, rashes, hemorrhoids, severe bruising, swelling, eczema, inflamed joints, muscle spasms, varicose veins, gum dis-ease, toothache, sore breasts, earache, eyestrain and inflammation, hair rinse; used in a steam kettle for asthma, hay fever, respiratory congestion; oil used as a chest rub for flu, colds; internal use for mucus conditions and congestion, respiratory viruses, colds, flu, children's infectious dis-eases such as chicken pox and measles, sinus infections and congestion; breaks fevers by inducing heavy sweating; internal use also for urinary tract for cystitis, urinary bleeding; digestive tonic and bitter that increases bile flow, reduces nausea, stimulates appetite; also used for diarrhea, dysentery, indigestion, gastritis, gas, and ulcers, including bleeding ulcers; tones the blood vessels and stops bleeding for nosebleeds, heavy menstruation, lung hemorrhage, and also reduces internal blood clots; for depression, emotional trauma, confusion, personality changes, headaches and migraines, high blood pressure, slowing heart rate (palpitations); contracts and tightens uterus, brings on menses, reduces menstrual pain, mastitis; leukemia cell suppression; promotes bone, muscle, and nerve growth and function, and aids physical coordination. *Astringent, anti-inflammatory, nerve tonic, stimulant, diuretic, stops bleeding, antiseptic, antibiotic.* Avoid overdose or prolonged use, especially in pregnancy (uterine stimulant); overdose side effects include allergic reactions, photosensitivity, and sperm count reduction in men; no known drug interactions.

Yellow Dock • (*Rumex crispus*)

Also called curly dock; purifies the blood, lymphatic system, and liver; for debility and deficiency when the body is too run-down to clear itself of toxins; high in accessible iron for people with iron deficiency, anemia, low red blood cell count, vegetarians with protein deficiency, debility from chemotherapy or radiation treatment, for women who hemorrhage severely with menstruation, and for those with tuberculosis, cancer, or other wasting or debilitating dis-eases; used externally

A
B
C
D
E
F
G
H
I
J
K
L
M
N
O
P
Q
R
S
T
U
V
W
X
Y
Z

(wash or salve) and internally for skin disorders: eczema, impetigo, thrush, itching of any kind, acne, boils, fungal infections, swelling, sores, scabby eruptions; strengthens liver function, increases liver's ability to store iron, detoxifies the liver, increases bile flow, clears jaundice, remedies sluggish digestion and constipation; nutritive support and tonic for pregnant women, and used for osteoarthritis and rheumatism. *Astringent, tonic, laxative.* Safe for long-term use in large doses; the only known side effect is diarrhea; no known drug interactions or warnings.

Yerba Mansa • *(Amenopsis californicum)*

Less endangered substitute for goldenseal, almost an all-healer; take with a lot of water because of its very bad taste; highly potent and strong, best saved for more serious conditions; use for all infections, especially chronic infections; acute or chronic sore throat and sores in the throat (internally and as a gargle), lung and sinus irritations; respiratory infections, bronchitis, flu especially long-term flu that won't go away, pneumonia, pleurisy, coughs; as a mouth rinse and internally for mouth sores, infections, and infected gums; as a wash for skin infections, wounds, rashes, and diaper rash; internally for colds, duodenal and stomach ulcers, intestinal diseases such as Crohn's dis-ease, ulcerative colitis, rheumatic dis-eases, arthritis, athlete's foot, infected wounds and sores (internally and externally), internal and external bleeding, urinary and kidney infections, cystitis, gout, diuretic, blood cleanser; as a douche for vaginal yeast infections, uterine dis-eases, and uterine cancer; in a sitz bath for hemorrhoids, after-childbirth healing, pelvic dis-eases, sexually tranmitted infections, and vaginal warts. *Anti-inflammatory, antifungal, antibacterial, antiviral, diuretic.* Possible diarrhea side effect, no known warnings or drug interactions.

Yerba Maté • *(Ilex paraguariensis)*
Caffeinated herbal tea from South America; high in nutrients, polyphenols, and saponins; used like green tea and brewed ritually; mental stimulant, study aid, increases alertness without anxiety or caffeine jitters, rejuvenates, reduces mental and physical fatigue, increases energy; antidepressant, stress reducer, muscle relaxant; tones the nervous system, reduces effects of debilitating dis-ease, aids insomnia;

A B C D E F G H I J K L M N O P Q R S T U V W X Y Z

antioxidant that protects the liver, DNA, and cells, lowers cholesterol; immune booster, strengthens resistance to dis-ease, accelerates healing; anticancer, antiaging, antibiotic, diuretic, digestive bitter; fights fungi, bacteria, microbes, and viruses; protects and stimulates heart function; promotes weight loss, laxative, colon cleanser; inhibits allergic reactions, hay fever, promotes sweating to break fevers, clears bad breath, balances high and low blood sugar levels. *Stimulant, bitter, nerve tonic, antioxidant, antiviral, astringent, diuretic, antibiotic.* Side effects include nausea, headache, nervousness, skin flushing, vomiting, irritability; not for use in pregnancy, while breast-feeding, for those with high blood pressure or liver dis-ease, or for children; caution with diabetes; no specifically listed drug interactions.

Yerba Santa • *(Eriodictyon californicum)*

Best known as an herbal decongestant and expectorant for upper respiratory viral dis-eases; breaks up mucus, expels phlegm, moisturizes and soothes congested and swollen mucous membranes; for colds, coughs, flu, sore throat, pleurisy, pneumonia, bronchitis, whooping cough, sinusitis, also asthma and chronic respiratory dis-eases, traditionally for tuberculosis; soothes digestion, increases salivation; digestive bitter; stimulates liver and stomach secretions, aids poor digestion with gas and fatigue, increases appetite, soothes stomachaches, diarrhea; used externally as a poultice or liniment to break fevers, for hemorrhoids, rheumatism, muscle fatigue, sprains, bruises, swelling, sores, boils, abscesses, acne, wounds, insect bites; dissolves warts; used with grindelia for poison ivy and poison oak; tones the nervous system, stimulates the mind, and relieves fatigue and exhaustion. *Antispasmodic, decongestant, expectorant, astringent, demulcent (lubricates), stimulant, antibacterial.* May cause side effects of insomnia or appetite loss; should not be used in pregnancy or while breastfeeding, or by those with chronic gastrointestinal dis-eases; caution with sleep disorders, insomnia, or with iron deficiency (may reduce iron absorption); no known drug interactions.

Yohimbe • *(Pausinystalia yohimbe)*

Included here as a warning, as there are more reasons not to take it than to take it; may be included in very small amounts in sexual enhancement combination remedies for men and occasionally for women; information below is for the single herb, which is not approved for legal use in the United States or Europe; used for sexual impotence and erectile dysfunction in men only; a male aphrodisiac and herbal Viagra; other uses for weight loss, body building, and depression have not proved valid or require too large amounts of the herb for safety; has a narrow therapeutic range—below it, there is no effect, and above it, the herb is dangerous; an MAO inhibitor (monoamine oxidase), users cannot eat tyramine-containing foods such as liver, aged cheese, and red wine, or use decongestants containing the drug phenylpropanolamine; causes dangerous rise in blood pressure, anxiety and panic attacks; overdose can be fatal; overdose effects include dangerously high blood pressure, seizures, hallucinations, paralysis, salivation, dilated pupils, irregular heartbeat, bowel evacuation, kidney failure, heart failure; normal dose side effects include dizziness, nausea, insomnia, anxiety, rapid heart rate, high blood pressure, tremors, headache, and agitation. In men with post-traumatic stress disorder, panic disorders, or Parkinson's disease, causes panic attacks and agitated anxiety; not for women or children; avoid with kidney dis-ease, liver dis-ease, ulcers heart dis-ease, high blood pressure, low blood pressure, panic disorders, posttraumatic stress disorder, or Parkinson's dis-ease; unsafe with blood pressure medication, alcohol, morphine, antidepressants, or any mood-altering drugs, including over-the-counter drugs.

Yucca • *(Yucca glauca, Yucca species)*

Also called soapwort and used as a soap by Native Americans of the Southwest; major actions of detoxification, anti-inflammatory, and natural cortisone; works like aspirin without aspirin side effects; beneficial for people and dogs; cleanser and purifier for blood, colon, kidneys, liver, gallbladder; digestive stimulant and general tonic; promising help for arthritis, joint pain and inflammation, bursitis, sprains, bone spurs, hip dysplasia in dogs; breaks up mineral deposits in the joints, promotes formation of healthy cartilage; improves digestion, reduces allergies, hot spots, skin disorders, itchy skin, bowel problems, colic; decreases swelling, stops bleeding, improves circulation, relieves pain; lowers blood pressure, LDL cholesterol, and blood sugar; may be antimelanoma and anticancer, provides support for Addison's dis-ease, balances positive flora in the gastrointestinal tract, reduces migraine frequency; used externally for hair loss and dandruff, skin lesions, sores, wounds, bleeding, and swelling; useful internally for rheumatism and gout, colitis, ulcers, sexually transmitted infections; laxative. *Anti-inflammatory, antibacterial, antifungal, tonic.* Mild possible side effects of nausea or diarrhea, long-term use can interfere with vitamin absorption; no known drug interactions.

ABOUT *the* AUTHOR

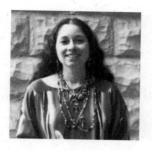

A healer for more than twenty-five years, DIANE STEIN is the best-selling author of *Essential Reiki* and more than twenty other books in the fields of metaphysics, women's spirituality, and alternative healing. She lives and teaches in Florida.

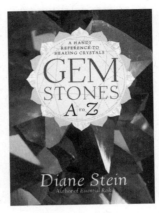